Practical Fluids
—and Electrolytes

Practical Fluids
—and Electrolytes—

John N. Krieger, MD
Professor of Urology
University of Washington School of Medicine
Seattle, Washington

Donald J. Sherrard, MD
Professor of Medicine/Nephrology
University of Washington School of Medicine
Chief, Nephrology
VA Medical Center
Seattle, Washington

with a Foreword by
Belding H. Scribner, MD
Professor of Medicine
University of Washington School of Medicine
Seattle, Washington

APPLETON & LANGE
Norwalk, Connecticut/San Mateo, California

0-8385-2621-7

 Copyright © 1991 by Appleton & Lange
A Publishing Division of Prentice Hall

91 92 93 94 95 / 10 9 8 7 6 5 4 3 2 1

Prentice Hall International (UK) Limited, *London*
Prentice Hall of Australia Pty. Limited, *Sydney*
Prentice Hall Canada, Inc., *Toronto*
Prentice Hall Hispanoamericana, S.A., *Mexico*
Prentice Hall of India Private Limited, *New Delhi*
Prentice Hall of Japan, Inc., *Tokyo*
Simon & Schuster Asia Pte. Ltd., *Singapore*
Editora Prentice Hall do Brasil Ltda., *Rio de Janeiro*
Prentice Hall, *Englewood Cliffs, New Jersey*

Library of Congress Cataloging-in-Publication Data
Krieger, John N.
  Practical fluids and electrolytes / John N. Krieger, Donald J. Sherrard.
    p. cm.
  Includes index.
  ISBN 0-8385-2621-7
  1. Water-electrolyte imbalances. 2. Acid-base imbalances.
  I. Sherrard, Donald J. II. Title.
  [DNLM: 1. Acid-Base Imbalance. 2. Kidney—physiology. 3. Water
  -Electrolyte Balance. 4. Water-Electrolyte Imbalance.   WD 220
  K92p]
  RC630.K75   1991
  616.3'9—dc20
  DNLM/DLC
  for Library of Congress   90-14481
                                                                    CIP

Acquisitions Editor: William R. Schmitt
Production Editors: Elizabeth Ryan, Susan Meiman
Designer: Janice Barsevich

PRINTED IN THE UNITED STATES OF AMERICA

Contents

Contributors

Suhail Ahmad, MD
Associate Professor of Medicine/Nephrology
University of Washington School of Medicine
Seattle, Washington

Ralph E. Cutler, MD
Professor of Medicine/Nephrology
Loma Linda University School of Medicine
Loma Linda, California

John N. Krieger, MD
Professor of Urology
University of Washington School of Medicine
Seattle, Washington

Donald J. Sherrard, MD
Professor of Medicine/Nephrology
University of Washington School of Medicine
Chief, Nephrology
VA Medical Center
Seattle, Washington

Preface

Understanding fluids, electrolytes, and acid-base disorders is one of the most difficult tasks facing students and clinicians. It is also one of the most essential. One major problem is that most textbooks are either difficult to understand, overly complicated, or irrelevant to problems encountered in clinical practice.

The goal of this book is to make this material as straightforward and understandable as possible. Fortunately, we have many years of experience teaching this subject in a variety of forums and to diverse audiences, including second-year medical students, nurses, physicians' assistants, clinical clerks, and our colleagues in practice. Based on this experience we have developed a practical and effective approach.

This book covers the basics, not the newest research. The underlying philosophy is that it is possible to present fundamental concepts in understandable and relatively painless fashion. Once that goal is accomplished, then the pathophysiology underlying major clinical disorders may be understood, not memorized.

The 13 chapters are organized into four sections. First, we consider basic renal physiology. Attention is then directed to normal fluid and electrolyte balance, emphasizing the role of the kidney. The third section covers the most common fluid and electrolyte disorders. The subjects include: body fluids and compartments, and the associated disorders of salt and water, potassium, and acid-base. The final section covers two important disorders, chronic renal failure and obstructive uropathy, that have specialized considerations for diagnosis and therapy.

Each chapter is accompanied by study questions and suggested answers to the questions. If you can answer the questions, then you don't need to read that chapter. The study questions serve two other purposes. First, they emphasize the major theoretical points of the chapter. Second, the questions often concern common clinical situations that require diagnosis and therapy. Placing these questions in juxtaposition to basic physiological concepts emphasizes the immediate clinical utility of our approach to fluid and electrolyte balance. If you understand the answers to the study questions, then you can correctly manage almost all patients with acid-base and fluid and electrolyte disorders.

The text is organized in outline format with numerous tables and illustrations. We have made a major effort to use boldface type for all important concepts. Thus, use of yellow markers should be unnecessary. Each chapter is designed to be read in 30 to 60 minutes and the entire book can be read in one or two weekends.

Foreword

During my fellowship at the Mayo Clinic, I published my first paper entitled *A Bedside Method for the Determination of Chloride*.[1] Since this method was rapid and simple and worked on all body fluids, including plasma, it became relatively easy to measure chloride balance on sick patients and calculate changes in the chloride space as an index of the patient's need for normal saline. A system for managing problems of fluid balance was devised based on this approach.[2]

In order to teach my colleagues at the Mayo Clinic how to use this approach to manage fluid balance problems, I put together a mimeographed pamphlet, which was the grandfather of the fluid balance sections in this volume. It is noteworthy that the principal component of that pamphlet has endured the test of time, and is an integral part of this volume. I refer to the two-step process of devising a daily plan of therapy by: (1) determination of **basic allowances**, and (2) modification of those allowances by adding or subtracting **corrections** in various categories, such as water, ECV, and acid-base. This format facilitates the logical application of knowledge to arrive at an individualized daily plan of fluid therapy, and is particularly useful in teaching this subject because it indicates to the instructor exactly what the student thinks is wrong with the patient. In addition, this format greatly facilitates the use of illustrative cases, which were an integral part of that original pamphlet and make this book uniquely valuable for teaching and understanding fluid balance.

When I moved to the University of Washington in 1951, the pamphlet came along and, with the help of numerous colleagues, gradually evolved into the *University of Washington Fluid Balance Syllabus*, which is the precursor of the fluid balance sections of this book. Of particular importance were the addition of the chapters on disorders of sodium and water balance and disorders of potassium balance, which were based on the publications of Burnell and Scribner.[3,4,5] This syllabus and its accompanying illustrative cases provided the basis for both undergraduate and postgraduate courses in fluid balance, which continue to the present time. Over the years it has been particularly rewarding to hear from former students how they quickly became fluid balance "experts" soon after starting internships in other institutions.

Our greatest mistake was never taking the time and making the effort to publish the fluid balance syllabus. So it is with great pleasure and satisfaction that I can congratulate the authors for finally getting the job done. I sincerely believe that as the subject is presented in this volume, together with the underlying renal physiology, it will make a unique contribution to the teaching and understanding of fluid and electrolyte balance.

Belding H. Scribner, MD
Professor of Medicine
University of Washington School of Medicine
Seattle, Washington

In 1960 Dr. Scribner was the first to initiate dialysis as the treatment for chronic renal failure.

References

1. Scribner BH: Bedside Determination of Chloride. *Proc Staff Meet Mayo Clin.* 1950; 25:641–645.
2. Scribner BH, Power MH, Rynearson EH: Bedside management of problems of fluid balance. *JAMA.* 1950; 144:1167–1174.
3. Burnell JM, Paton RR, Scribner BH: The problem of sodium and water needs of patients. *J Chron Dis.* 1960; 11:189–198.
4. Scribner BH, Burnell JM: Interpretation of the serum potassium concentration. *Metabolism.* 1956; 5:468–479.
5. Burnell JM, Villamil M, Uyeno B, Scribner BH: The effect in humans of extracellular pH change on the relationship between serum potassium concentration and intracellular potassium. *J Clin Invest.* 1956; 35:935–989.

Functions and Structure of the Urinary System

INTRODUCTION

Consideration of fluids and electrolytes must begin with a review of the urinary system, as this is the primary organ system. This chapter discusses the structure and functions of the urinary system, emphasizing renal physiology. In addition, some of the major developmental abnormalities of the kidney, as well as the urinary drainage system, are examined.

STUDY QUESTIONS

1. Summarize the functions of the urinary system.
2. List 10 major developmental abnormalities of the kidney.
3. Briefly describe any 5 of the conditions in Question 2.
4. Describe the blood supply of the kidney.
5. List the major components of the nephron and briefly describe the function of each structure (maximum of one statement per structure).

FUNCTIONS OF THE URINARY SYSTEM

Why Do We Have A Urinary System?

The answer to this question lies in the workings of the individual cells. Millions of **intracellular chemical reactions depend on the concentrations of both intracellular ions and water**. The optimum environment for these reactions is maintained by active transport processes plus selective permeability of the cell membrane, which can tolerate slight variations in the extracellular environment. However, intracellular transport processes cannot cope with wide fluctuations in the extracellular environment. Such changes may alter intracellular composition sufficiently to impair metabolic activity and may even cause irreversible damage or death.

Higher animals can function only because their cells are not exposed directly to the widely fluctuating environment. The immediate environment of individual cells is called the extracellular fluid or the internal environment. **Conditions in the extracellular fluid are remarkably constant despite the wide fluctuations in the external environment.** This constancy of the internal environment, or **homeostasis,** is achieved by sophisticated regulatory and excretory processes involving the cardiovascular, respiratory, and urinary systems. These systems, in turn, are controlled by complex neural and hormonal mechanisms.

The specific role of the urinary system is to maintain the proper extracellular fluid volume and the proper concentrations of the fixed (nonvolatile) solutes.

Renal Regulation of the Internal Environment

The Balance Concept. A substance can appear in the body only as the result of ingestion or of metabolism. Conversely, a substance can only be excreted from the body or consumed in a metabolic reaction. Therefore, if the quantity of any substance in the body is to be maintained at a constant level over time, **the total amounts ingested and produced must equal the total amounts excreted and consumed.** This is a general statement of the balance concept.

For water and hydrogen ion, also known as hydrion, all four possible pathways occur. These substances appear in the body as the result of both ingestion and metabolism, and they are both excreted from the body and consumed in metabolic reactions. The balance concept is simpler for mineral electrolytes. Since they are neither synthesized nor consumed by cells, their total body balance reflects only ingestion and excretion.

Overview of Kidney Functions. The kidney has three major functions: (1) **regulation of the internal environment**, (2) **excretion of by-products of metabolism**, and (3) **endocrine functions.** The kidney has a major regulatory function as the primary organ responsible for controlling the properties and balance of most ions in the extracellular fluid. In addition to this regulatory role, the kidneys function as major organs for elimination of the end products of metabolism. Finally, the kidneys function as endocrine organs, producing substances, such as erythropoietin (critical for maintaining red blood cell mass), and renin (important in control of blood pressure) and activating vitamin D (important in calcium metabolism).

Functions of the Collecting and Voiding System. The collecting and voiding system is composed of the renal pelves, ureters, urinary bladder, and urethra. The function of the collecting system is **to transport urine from the kidney to the bladder while keeping the renal pelvic pressure low and maintaining a sterile urine. In the bladder, urine is stored until a suitable time and place occur for evacuation.**

The urinary tract is lined by transitional epithelium from the renal papilla to a variable point in the distal urethra. These cells allow an insignificant net exchange of ions and water, maintaining urinary composition as determined by the kidney. The transitional epithelium can adapt to rapid changes in surface area, an important property for normal bladder function.

ANATOMY OF THE URINARY SYSTEM

Development of the Kidney
The development of the urinary system follows a sequence of changes that involve **replacement of the original kidney by a second kidney, then replacement of this system by a third kidney. In contrast, the original ducts that drain these systems undergo modification rather than replacement.** Portions of this evolving duct system may be discarded or incorporated into the reproductive system. This accounts for the brief association between the urinary and reproductive systems in the female and the persistent association of these systems in the male.

The **pronephros is the first kidney.** Although it is functional in certain primitive fishes and in amphibian larvae, it makes only a transitory appearance in embryonic birds and mammals. In humans, the pronephros never becomes functional.

The **mesonephros** is the adult kidney of fishes and amphibia. It appears in the human embryo during the fourth week of gestation, then degenerates. **Mesonephric remnants play a role in the reproductive system, and the mesonephric**

duct is important in development of the collecting system of the kidney. The ureteric bud originates from the mesonephric duct and subsequently gives rise to the renal pelvis, calyces, papillary ducts, and collecting tubules.

The **metanephros** is the definitive kidney in mammals. It **provides the functioning kidney** down to the distal tubules. At this point, the metanephros fuses with the ureteric bud (a structure derived from the mesonephric duct). The metanephros is the final kidney in humans. Description of its function is the subject of this book.

Congenital Anomalies of the Kidney

Developmental abnormalities affect the genitourinary system more frequently than any other organ system. Development of normal renal architecture may be disrupted by three types of developmental abnormalities: anomalies of size and number, anomalies of location, and cystic diseases.

Anomalies of Size and Number

Agenesis. **Complete absence of renal development** is termed renal agenesis. This process may affect one or both kidneys. Bilateral renal agenesis is the most extreme developmental abnormality. Because there is no function of the developing kidneys, bilateral renal agenesis is associated with markedly reduced amounts of amniotic fluid (termed oligohydramnios). The lungs do not develop, since the developing embryo must inhale the amniotic fluid to ensure normal pulmonary development. Bilateral renal agenesis is a rare and uniformly **fatal** abnormality.

Solitary Kidney. **Solitary kidney** (unilateral renal agenesis) occurs in approximately 1 of 500 people. This condition is **usually asymptomatic.** Clinical discovery occurs as the result of diagnostic evaluation for other conditions. The surviving kidney is usually enlarged, a process known as **compensatory hypertrophy.**

Duplications. **Duplications of the renal pelvis and collecting system are common.** Up to 10% of individuals have some degree of duplication. This may be minimal or may include complete duplication of the renal pelvis and ureter.

Anomalies of Location. Ectopic kidney is the term used to describe an abnormality in location of the kidney. This abnormality occurs slightly less frequently than solitary kidney.

Simple Ectopia. **Simple ectopia** is malposition of a kidney located on the normal side. The most frequent location is in the bony pelvis, and this condition is termed **pelvic kidney.** Pelvic kidneys often can be palpated and have been removed by unwary surgeons following the incorrect diagnosis of a retroperitoneal tumor.

Crossed Ectopia. **Crossed ectopia** occurs when a kidney with a ureter from one side crosses the midline to the **other side.** Because of abnormal rotation and location, these kidneys are particularly susceptible to obstruction.

Horseshoe Kidney. **Horseshoe kidneys** occur with a frequency of 1 per 400 to 700 live births. In this anomaly, the two **kidneys are fused,** usually at the lower pole, leading to formation of a horseshoe-shaped mass of renal tissue. The kidney mass is fused anterior to the aorta. This condition is clinically significant because the fused kidneys do not rotate normally during development due to fixation of each kidney to its counterpart on the other side. This means that the renal pelvis drains anteriorly over the isthmus of the horseshoe kidney (compared to the unobstructed, dependent drainage of the normal kidney). Thus, horseshoe kidneys usually are diagnosed because of the effects of **obstruction, infection, or stone formation.** These kidneys often have multiple abnormalities in their vascular supply, with multiple renal arteries arising from the aorta and other major vessels.

Cystic Diseases. Such conditions often represent **abnormalities in the process by which the ureteric bud contacts the developing metanephros.**

Polycystic Kidney Disease. These patients have inherited renal failure due to the presence of a multitude of cysts within the kidneys. There are two clinical types of polycystic disease: an adult type and a childhood type.

    Adult polycystic kidney disease. The adult form of polycystic renal disease is inherited as a simple **autosomal dominant** with high penetrance. The **kidneys are huge,** often filling both flanks and extending into the lower abdomen. Individual cysts may be barely visible or up to 5 cm in diameter. They are filled with clear, straw-colored fluid. Approximately one third of the patients with this disease have associated cysts of the liver, and 15% have cerebral artery aneurysms (which cause death in 10%). Most patients develop symptoms during their fourth decade, with **renal failure at about 50 years old.** Common symptoms include a feeling of fullness in the flanks, flank masses, hypertension, and hematuria.

    Infantile polycystic disease. The infantile form of polycystic disease is rare. The cysts are smaller than those in the adult form, but the kidneys are enlarged and occasionally interfere with delivery. Almost all patients **die in the perinatal period.** The usual cause of death is respiratory failure as a result of the huge renal masses interfering with normal pulmonary expansion.

Cystic Conditions of the Medulla. There are two important cystic conditions that occur in the renal medulla, medullary sponge kidney and medullary cystic disease.

    Medullary sponge kidney consists of tubular **dilation of the collecting ducts.** The cystic dilations commonly are associated with stones and infections but, fortunately, not with renal failure. The condition is more common in males than in females.

    Medullary cystic disease causes renal failure in young patients. There is some familial tendency, and renal failure usually develops in the first two decades. Most patients have anemia, which is a consequence of their renal failure (uremia).

Simple Renal Cysts. These cysts are very common. It is estimated that half of the population over the age of 50 has simple renal cysts. Most simple cysts are asymptomatic, and they rarely interfere with renal function. On occasion, a simple cyst may cause symptoms because of rupture, infection, or hemorrhage. Simple cysts are primarily important in the differential diagnosis of a renal mass lesion, a situation in which cyst must be distinguished from renal cancer.

Renal Dysplasia. Renal dysplasia is a general term used to describe **abnormalities in development and organization of the kidney.** Renal dysplasia is the most common cystic disorder in pediatric patients. Dysplasia is also the **most frequent cause of a renal mass in the newborn.** Clinically, the only manifestation of this disease is the presence of a mass. Grossly, the dysplastic kidney is a clump of cysts, often resembling a bunch of grapes, with little resemblance to a normal kidney. Prognosis in patients with unilateral dysplasia is excellent because normal function of the opposite kidney is sufficient for normal growth and development. The rare occurrence of bllateral renal dysplasia is not compatible with life.

Gross Anatomy

Beginning from the upper (cranial) end of the urinary tract, urine is made in the kidneys, then passes sequentially through the renal pelves, ureters, and bladder, and finally is excreted through the urethra.

Kidneys

Location. The kidneys are located in the dorsal part of the abdomen, one on either side of the vertebral column (Fig. 1–1). The upper renal margin is at the level of the 12th thoracic vertebra, and the lower margin extends to the 3rd lumbar vertebra. The **kidneys lie in the retroperitoneum,** that is, the portion of the abdominal cavity that is posterior to the posterior parietal peritoneum covering the intraabdominal organs. A layer of fat, termed the **perirenal fat, immediately surrounds the kidneys and is contained within the perirenal fascia** (commonly known as **Gerota's fascia**). The kidney parenchyma is covered by a fibrous capsule. Since they are in contact with the diaphragm, the kidneys move with respiration.

Major Components. The normal adult kidney is about 11.5 cm long, 5 to 7 cm wide, and 2.5 cm thick. It weighs about 115 to 155 g in females and 125 to 170 g in males. The major renal components are

- Parenchyma
    Medulla
    Cortex
- Collecting system
    Calix
    Pelvis
    Ureter

  The kidney is composed of the parenchyma and the collecting system. The parenchyma **filters and modifies the urine.** The collecting system transports the

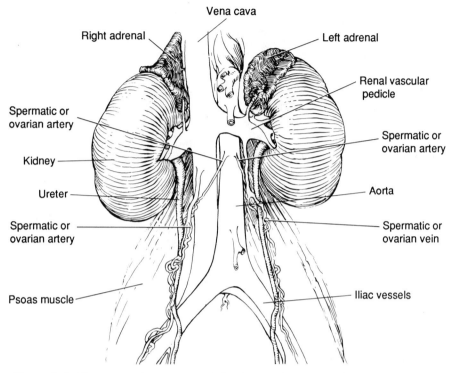

Figure 1–1. The upper urinary tract is similar in the male and female (anteroposterior view). (*Modified from Tanagho EA, McAninch JW: Smith's General Urology, 12th ed. Norwalk, Conn: Appleton & Lange, 1988, p. 2.*)

urine. The **renal parenchyma is composed of an inner medullary portion and an outer cortical portion** (Fig. 1–2). The renal medulla consists of 8 to 18 conical pyramids. The cortex extends from the medulla to the renal capsule. The cortical substance arches over the bases of the medullary pyramids and extends between adjacent pyramids to form the **renal columns.**

The **renal hilum** is located at the medial aspect of each kidney and is the point where the kidney **receives the blood and lymphatic vessels, ureter, and nerves.** This central area also contains the renal collecting system. The **collecting system is composed of the calyces, renal pelvis, and ureter.** These structures function to **transport the urine.** The renal pyramids indent the minor calices. There are usually 8 to 12 minor calices, which join to form 2 to 3 major calices. The major calices in turn unite to form the renal pelvis. The renal pelvis drains into the ureter, which, in turn, connects the kidney to the bladder.

Blood and Lymphatic Supply. **The renal artery arises directly from the aorta.** The main renal artery divides into two trunks, the anterior and posterior divisions. These branch to form the segmental arteries. There are five **segmental arteries.** Each is an end artery, similar to the coronary arteries. Thus, blockage of a seg-

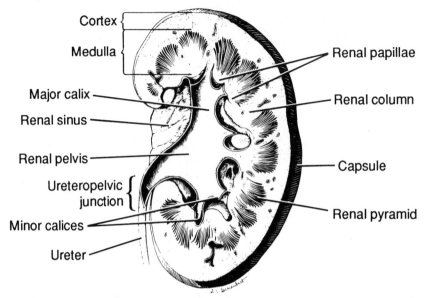

Cortex
Medulla
Major calix
Renal sinus
Renal pelvis
Ureteropelvic junction
Minor calices
Ureter
Renal papillae
Renal column
Capsule
Renal pyramid

Figure 1–2. The kidney in cross section (posterior view). (*Modified from Lindner HH: Clinical Anatomy. Norwalk, Conn: Appleton & Lange, 1989, p. 444.*)

mental artery leads to ischemia and death of a particular vascular segment. The segmental arteries divide sequentially into interlobar, arcuate, and interlobular vessels. The **interlobular vessels supply the glomeruli via the afferent arterioles.**

Venous return occurs via the **main renal vein,** which **drains into the vena cava.** In contrast to the renal arterial supply, there are anastomotic connections within the intrarenal venous network.

Lymphatics of the kidney drain into the hilar nodes, then into the lumbar lymph nodes. The **renal pelvis drains into the ureter at the ureteropelvic junction.**

Ureters. The ureter is a tubular structure that is about 30 cm long in the adult. The ureters are divided into three regions, abdominal, iliac, and pelvic (Fig. 1–1). Each section of the ureter has a narrow area: (1) **the ureteropelvic junction, where the renal pelvis drains into the ureter,** (2) the point where the ureter crosses the iliac vessels, and (3) the **ureterovesical junction, where the ureter enters the bladder.** These narrow areas are the points where calculi tend to become impacted. From the inside out, the ureter is composed of three layers, mucosa, muscularis, and adventitia.

The renal arteries supply the calyces, pelvis, and upper ureter. The midureter is supplied by the lumbar and gonadal arteries. At this point, the blood supply is most tenuous, and the ureter is especially susceptible to trauma or iatrogenic injury. The lower ureter receives its blood supply from the common iliac, hypogastric, and vesical arteries. Venous drainage is paired with the arteries.

Bladder. The urinary bladder is a musculomembranous sac that serves as a reservoir for urine. Its size and position vary according to the amount of fluid it contains. When moderately full, the bladder contains about 500 mL and assumes an oval shape. On its interior surface, the **trigone is delineated by the openings of the ureters and the urethra.** The interureteric ridge extends between the ureteral orifices.

Urethra. The urethra is the terminal segment of the urinary tract. There are marked differences between the normal female and male urethral anatomy.

Female. The female urethra is about 4 cm long (Fig. 1–3). It courses beneath the symphysis pubis anterior to the vagina. Opening is controlled by both an internal, smooth muscle (involuntary) sphincter and an external, striated muscle (voluntary) sphincter. The female urethra is lined by stratified squamous epithelium.

Male. Three regions of the male urethra are identified, the prostatic urethra, the membranous urethra, and the cavernous (spongy) urethra (Fig. 1–4). The **prostatic urethra** is approximately 3 cm long. The prostate and paired ejaculatory ducts

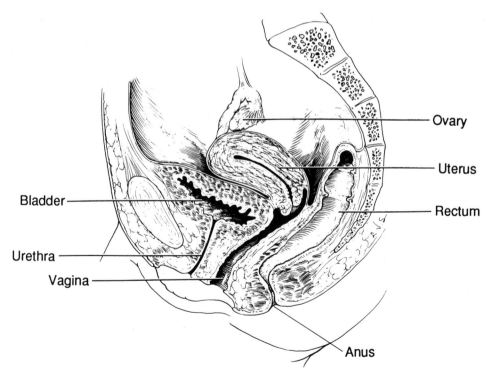

Figure 1–3. Lower genitourinary tract in the female (cross section). (*Modified from Tanagho EA, McAninch JW: Smith's General Urology, 12th ed. Norwalk, Conn: Appleton & Lange, 1988, p. 22.*)

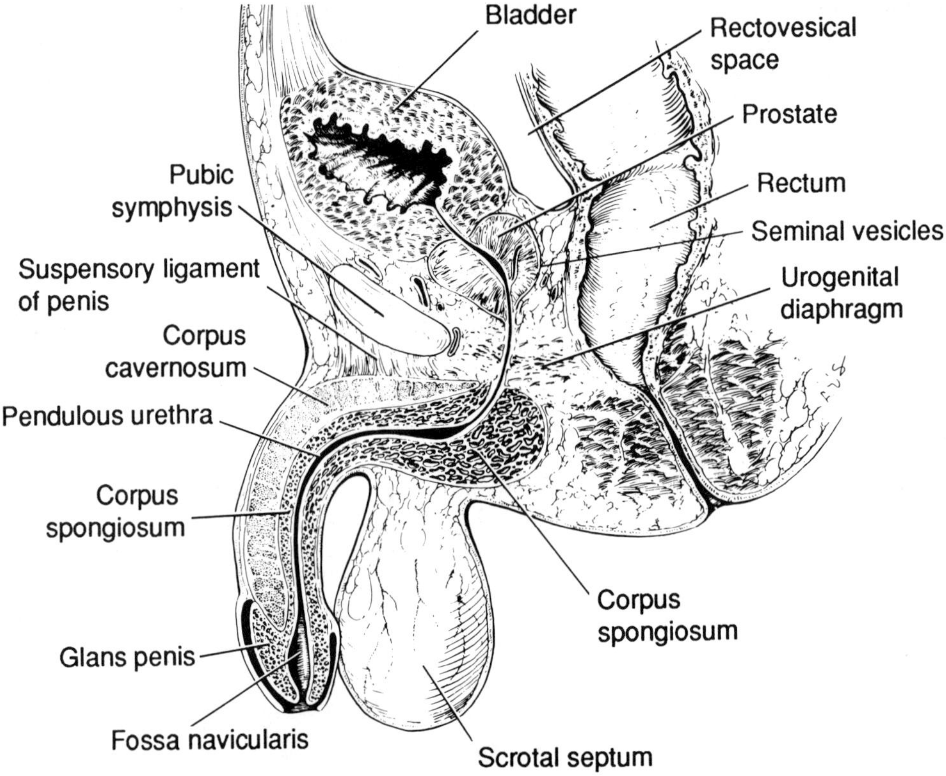

Figure 1–4. Lower urinary tract in the male (cross section). (*Modified from Tanagho EA, McAninch JW: Smith's General Urology, 12th ed. Norwalk, Conn: Appleton & Lange, 1988, p. 20.*)

(originating from the seminal vesicles) drain into the prostatic urethra. The **membranous urethra** is the shortest segment, only 2.5 cm long, and it contains the external, striated muscular sphincter. The longest segment is the **cavernous urethra,** which is approximately 15 cm long and terminates at the urethral meatus.

Microscopic Anatomy of the Kidney

General Structure. **The cut surface of the kidney reveals a cortex and medulla. The medulla consists of pyramids whose apices (papillae) fit into minor calyces. Medullary rays (straight tubules) extend from the base of the pyramids into the cortex. Cortical renal columns extend between the pyramids. A lobe consists of an overlying pyramid and cortex. A lobule includes a medullary ray (a bundle of straight tubules plus all the associated nephrons). A single lobe contains several lobules.**

Uriniferous Tubules. **Uriniferous tubules consist of nephrons and their collecting system.** Both of these have elements in the cortex and the medulla.

Nephron. The nephron is the star character in this book. Thus, we describe it in some detail. Each kidney contains about 1 to 2 million **functional units** called nephrons. **The nephron consists of groups of specialized cells that filter the blood, then selectively modify the filtrate by reabsorption or secretion of a variety of substances.** Each nephron is composed of four sections: the renal corpuscle, the proximal convoluted tubule, the loop of Henle, and the distal convoluted tubule (Fig. 1–5).

Renal Corpuscle. The renal corpuscle **consists of a glomerulus plus Bowman's capsule. The glomerulus (capillary tuft) has an afferent (arriving) and an efferent (exiting) arteriole.**

Bowman's capsule is a double-walled cup surrounding the glomerulus. Ultrastructural studies have demonstrated that the inner (visceral) layer of this cup consists of a specialized epithelium composed of podocytes, whose cytoplasmic

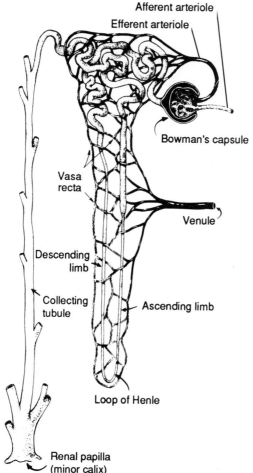

Figure 1–5. The nephron. *(Modified from Tanagho EA, McAninch JW: Smith's General Urology, 12th ed. Norwalk, Conn: Appleton & Lange, 1988, p. 5.)*

projections (foot processes) are directed toward the walls of glomerular capillaries. The visceral layer of Bowman's capsule is continuous with the parietal layer (simple squamous epithelium) at the vascular pole. Together, **these two layers of Bowman's capsule define the urinary space.**

The cells of the glomerular capillaries and those of the visceral layer of Bowman's capsule combine to form the glomerular filter. Components of this filter include

1. Endothelial pores or fenestrations, which are too small to allow passage of blood cells
2. Basal lamina, or basement membrane, a combination of fine collagen filaments and ground substance; this layer impedes passage of large molecules, especially albumin
3. Pores, or filtration slits, the smallest opening in the barrier, which prevent passage of molecules $\geq$ 100,000 daltons

Tubules. Generally, the renal tubules follow a winding route in the cortex (proximal and distal convoluted tubules) and a straight one in the medulla (**loop of Henle**). The loop of Henle is composed of the straight portion of the proximal tubule, the thin segment, and the straight portion of the distal tubule.

PROXIMAL, CONVOLUTED, AND THICK DESCENDING STRAIGHT TUBULES. The tubule walls are composed of a cuboidal to pyramidal epithelium with characteristic **ultrastructural features indicating a large capacity for metabolic activity.** The cells display brush borders (large absorptive surface), apical canaliculi (site of protein uptake), lysosomes (intracellular protein digestion), abundant mitochondria, and extensive infoldings of lateral and basal plasma membranes (large transport capacity).

The proximal tubules **reabsorb most of the filtrate.** Pumps in the plasma membrane actively reabsorb sodium, potassium, amino acids, and glucose. Water and urea are reabsorbed passively. Organic acids and bases are secreted actively, and proteins are reabsorbed by pinocytosis (vesicular transport).

THIN DESCENDING STRAIGHT TUBULE. The appearance of this portion of the nephron indicates **minimal specialization of the cells for active transport processes.** The thin segment has a low epithelium with no brush border. Adjacent cells interdigitate their lateral plasma membranes. The length of the thin descending straight tubule depends on the location of its glomerulus. Cortical glomeruli have short thin segments, whereas juxtamedullary glomeruli have long thin segments.

The tubule wall is **permeable** to the movements of urea, water, and sodium chloride. The **tubular fluid (filtrate) equilibrates with the ever-increasing osmolality of the interstitial fluid** as it flows toward the papilla through the loop of Henle.

THIN AND THICK COMPONENTS OF THE ASCENDING TUBULAR STRUCTURE. The appearance of the thin ascending tubule resembles that of the descending tubule. The thick portion is lined by a cuboidal epithelium, and the cells display an abundance of mitochondria and basal infoldings of the plasma membrane. In contrast to the thick descending tubule, there is no brush border—simply a few scattered microvilli on the cell apex.

Epithelial cells lining the thick and thin segments actively transport sodium chloride from the tubular lumen (filtrate) into the interstitium. Because the ascending tubule is poorly permeable to water, water cannot follow sodium chloride into the interstitial space. Therefore, the urine becomes dilute.

The unique looping characteristics of these segments and the vasa recta plus their special transport characteristics produce a **progressive increase in the interstitial osmolality from the cortex to the papillary tip.** This feature **is critical for both concentration and dilution of urine.**

DISTAL CONVOLUTED TUBULES. These cells resemble those of the ascending thick segment. The thick segment of the ascending tubule returns to the glomerulus with which it is in continuity.

Sodium is transported actively from the tubular lumen into the interstitium. Potassium and hydrogen ions are secreted into the urine. Because the epithelium is **impermeable to water,** the **urine remains dilute** in this segment.

COLLECTING TUBULES. **Final concentration of the urine** occurs in the medullary collecting tubules. **Antidiuretic hormone (ADH) increases the permeability of the collecting duct to water, enabling it to diffuse toward the hypertonic interstitial space.** Movement of water out of the tubule and into the interstitial space concentrates the urine. The net effect is to retain water. In the absence of ADH, the collecting tubules are poorly permeable to water, and a dilute urine is excreted.

Interstitium. The interstitium, or interstitial space, is the fluid-containing space surrounding the nephrons. **Differences in the osmotic concentrations of the fluid in the interstitial space, filtrate, and blood are maintained by the countercurrent exchange and multiplier systems** described in Chapter 5.

Capillary Blood Supply of the Tubules

Peritubular Capillaries. Efferent arterioles draining the superficial cortical glomeruli break up into capillaries that generally supply tubules of the same nephron before draining into the renal veins. On the other hand, the capillaries of the midcortex and the juxtaglomerular nephrons may supply a number of different nephrons.

Vasa Recta. Capillaries from efferent arterioles of the juxtamedullary glomeruli drain into a network of vessels that form the vasa recta. These hairpin loops course into the medullary pyramid toward the tip of the papilla alongside the loops of Henle.

Juxtaglomerular Apparatus. The juxtaglomerular apparatus consists of three parts: the juxtaglomerular (JG) cells, the macula densa, a modification of the distal tubule, and mesangial cells, which occupy the space between the afferent and efferent arterioles.

The JG cells are the most important element. JG cells are modified smooth muscle cells that have cytoplasmic granules containing the enzyme, renin. The **JG cells release renin** into the blood, initiating a series of reactions. This leads to production of angiotensin II, an octapeptide **having a major effect on blood pressure and electrolyte balance.**

SAMPLE ANSWERS TO STUDY QUESTIONS

1. Summarize the functions of the urinary system.

The urinary system maintains homeostasis in the extracellular fluid despite wide fluctuations in the external environment. It maintains proper extracellular fluid volume and concentrations of fixed solutes.

There are two major components of the urinary system: (1) the kidney and (2) the collecting and voiding system. Kidney functions include regulation of the internal environment, excretion of the by-products of metabolism, and endocrine functions. Collecting and voiding system functions include transport of urine to the bladder, and storage of urine in the bladder until a suitable time and place occur for evacuation.

2. List 10 major developmental abnormalities of the kidney.

1. Bilateral agenesis
2. Solitary kidney
3. Duplication of the collecting system
4. Simple ectopia
5. Crossed ectopia
6. Horseshoe kidney
7. Adult polycystic disease
8. Infantile polycystic disease
9. Medullary sponge kidney
10. Medullary cystic disease

3. Briefly describe any 5 of the conditions in Question 2.

Bilateral renal agenesis is complete absence of renal development. This condition is incompatible with life.

Solitary kidney is known also as unilateral renal agenesis. The patient has renal tissue only on one side and has half the normal number of nephrons. This condition is usually asymptomatic, and there is usually compensatory hypertrophy of the functioning kidney.

Simple ectopia is malposition of the kidney located on the normal side. The most common position is in the pelvis, a condition known as pelvic kidney.

Crossed ectopia is malposition of the kidney, with the kidney located on the opposite side. These kidneys are especially susceptible to obstruction because they are malrotated.

Renal dysplasia is an abnormality in development and organization of the kidney. This is the most common cause of a renal mass in the neonate.

4. Describe the blood supply of the kidney.

The renal artery is a direct branch of the aorta. It divides into anterior and posterior divisions, which give rise to five segmental arteries. The segmental arteries divide to become eventually the afferent (entering) and efferent (exiting) vessels supplying the glomeruli. The segmental arteries of the kidney are end arteries, which means that disruption of these vessels leads to infarction of the portion of the kidney supplied by that vessel. Venous return occurs by the main renal vein, which drains into the vena cava.

5. List the major components of the nephron and briefly describe the function of each structure (maximum of one statement per structure).

This is answered as Table 1–1.

TABLE 1–1. THE NEPHRON

Major Component	Function
Renal corpuscle	
Glomerulus	The filter
Bowman's capsule	Defines urinary space and contains filtrate
Tubules	
proximal, convoluted, and thick descending straight	Reabsorb most of the filtrate
Thin descending straight	Filtrate equilibrates with hypertonic interstitium
Thin and thick ascending	Active sodium chloride reabsorption without water reabsorption
Distal convoluted	Ion reabsorption and secretion
Collecting tubules	Final adjustment of urine osmolar and electrolyte composition

Renal Blood Flow and Glomerular Filtration

INTRODUCTION

Maintenance of the internal milieu is the most important function of the kidney.
This is accomplished by constant filtration of a large volume of plasma (180 L/
day), followed by appropriate modification of the ultrafiltrate, so that what is

needed by the body is retained and what is extra, or harmful, is excreted. To fulfill this task, **the kidney needs a large and uninterrupted supply of blood.**

First, the total amount of blood going to the kidney must be sufficient to produce large volumes of filtrate. This means a lot of blood. In fact, **the kidneys require approximately 25% of the total cardiac output.**

Second, **the blood supply to the kidneys must be maintained constant**, despite the normal fluctuations in arterial pressures. Because the systemic arterial pressure varies widely, the renal blood flow needs to be protected from these fluctuations. In normal persons, the renal blood flow is regulated to fulfill both of these requirements.

STUDY QUESTIONS

1. **a.** How much plasma flows through normal adult kidneys in 1 day?
   b. Why is such a large plasma volume needed by the kidneys?
2. **a.** Define the filtration fraction (FF).
   b. If the FF is 30% and renal plasma flow (RPF) is 660 mL/min, is the glomerular filtration rate (GFR) normal, subnormal, or higher than normal?
3. **a.** Name the major sites of renal resistance.
   b. What is the significance of afferent and efferent arteriolar pressure?
4. **a.** What is autoregulation, and why is it important?
   b. In what pressure range is autoregulation operative?
5. **a.** What happens to GFR if afferent arteriolar resistance increases?
   b. What happens if efferent arteriolar resistance increases?
6. If the para-aminohippurate (PAH) concentration in blood is high (> 15 mg/dL), would PAH clearance be equal to, less than, or greater than renal plasma flow (RPF)?
7. From the data given, calculate the renal clearance of (a) inulin, (b) urea, and (c) para-aminohippurate (PAH).

   $[\text{inulin}]_u$ = 100 mg/dL
   $[\text{inulin}]_p$ = 1 mg/dL
   $[\text{urea}]_u$ = 220 mmol/L
   $[\text{urea}]_p$ = 5 mmol/L
   $[\text{PAH}]_u$ = 1000 mg/dL
   $[\text{PAH}]_p$ = 2 mg/dL

RENAL BLOOD FLOW AND ANATOMY

Normal Renal Blood Flow

The weight of the kidney is similar to that of the heart, but the **renal blood flow (RBF) is over four times greater than the coronary circulation.** Plasma is filtered in the glomerular part of the nephron. The glomeruli are located in the outer portion of the **kidney, termed the renal cortex. In normal adults, the renal blood flow (RBF) is 1200 mL/min.** Therefore, with a hematocrit of 45%, the **renal plasma**

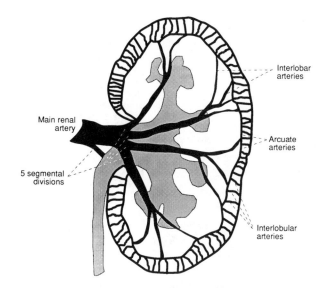

Figure 2–1. The renal arterial supply (anterior schematic view).

flow (RPF) is 660 mL/min. * About 90% of RBF is directed to the renal cortex, and the remaining 10% is directed to the medulla. Any marked reduction in RPF results in reduction in the glomerular filtration rate (GFR).

Pertinent Renal Anatomy

The renal artery divides sequentially into segmental branches, interlobar arteries, arcuate arteries, interlobular arteries, then afferent arterioles (Fig. 2–1). **The afferent arterioles supply the glomerular capillaries.** The blood plasma is filtered across the glomerular capillary membranes. The glomerular capillaries rejoin to form **efferent arterioles through which blood exits out of the glomeruli.**

There are three main sites of resistance that adjust the hydrostatic pressure in the kidney: the afferent arteriole, the efferent arteriole, and the venules (Fig. 2–2). The afferent arteriole is the first and the main site** of resistance. At this site, the pressure drops to 50 torr from a systemic mean arterial pressure of 100 torr. The second site of resistance is the efferent arteriole, where there is a further drop in pressure to 15 to 20 torr in the peritubular capillaries.

Thus, the **intraglomerular pressure is maintained at about 50 torr by the interplay of the afferent and efferent arteriolar resistance.** This constant intraglomerular pressure is maintained even **in the presence of fluctuating systemic pressure.** Maintenance of a stable intraglomerular pressure **ensures a constant GFR (autoregulation).**

The relatively **lower pressure in the peritubular capillaries favors reabsorption** of the tubular fluid. The third site of resistance is at the level of the venules,

---

*Since hematocrit = RBC volume = 45%
   blood volume − RBC volume = plasma volume
   plasma volume = 55% of blood volume
   RBF = 1200 mL/min
Therefore, normal RPF = 0.55 (1200 mL/min) = 660 mL/min.

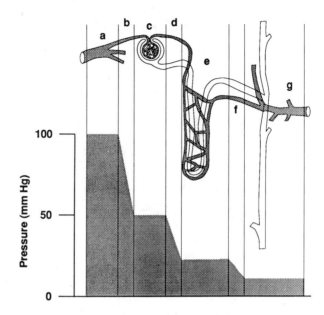

Figure 2–2. Resistance sites along the renal vasculature. **a.** Renal artery. **b.** Afferent arteriole. **c.** Glomerulus. **d.** Efferent arteriole. **e.** Peritubular capillaries. **f.** Venule. **g.** Renal vein. *(From Knox FG (ed): Textbook of Renal Patho-physiology, Hagerstown, MD: Harper and Row, 1978, p. 75.)*

which protects the renal capillaries from fluctuations in the central venous pressure.

GLOMERULAR FILTRATION

Definition
Filtration is the flow of a solvent through a porous barrier. The solvent carries any solutes that are small enough to pass through the pores of the filter. The glomeruli behave qualitatively like other capillaries by allowing passage of water and electrolytes, as well as small organic molecules, such as glucose, while retaining large solutes, such as plasma proteins and macromolecules.

Factors Important in the Filtration Process

Surface Area. **The large surface area and high permeability of glomerular capillaries favor filtration.** The total surface area of glomeruli is estimated to be about 1.6 m², an area nearly as large as the total body surface area of the average adult. Filtration through this capillary bed is enhanced by the relatively large fraction of the surface that is available for filtration, 2 to 3% of glomerular capillary surface, compared with only 0.1% of muscle capillaries. In addition, glomerular capillaries are immensely more permeable to water and small solutes than are muscle capillaries. The large filtration surface and high permeability produce a huge **glomerular filtrate of approximately 180 L/day** in the adult.

   This large volume of fluid undergoes extensive modification as it flows down the tubules to become urine. Furthermore, from knowledge of your own rate of urine excretion, it should be obvious that about **99% of the glomerular filtrate is reabsorbed.** Lack of tubular reabsorption would lead to dangerous depletion of body fluids in 1 to 2 hours.

The Filtration Barrier. The filtration barrier is not homogeneous. It consists of a series of complex structures that collectively determine the kinds of particles that cross the capillary wall (Fig. 2–3). The filtration barrier is composed of three major anatomic components: the capillary endothelium, the basement membrane, and the pedicle layer of the podocytes.

Capillary Endothelium. For a molecule to enter Bowman's space from the capillary lumen, it must first traverse the capillary endothelium (Fig. 2–3). The endothelium presents little impediment to filtration because large molecules (450,000 daltons) move through the endothelial pores, which are larger and more irregular than in other fenestrated capillaries.

Basement Membrane. The next barrier encountered is the basement membrane. It is currently thought that the basement membrane, consisting mostly of type IV collagen, is **the most significant part of the glomerular filter.**

Podocyte Foot Processes. The final barrier is the foot process layer of the podocytes, bridged by the filtration slit membrane. In general, neutral molecules smaller

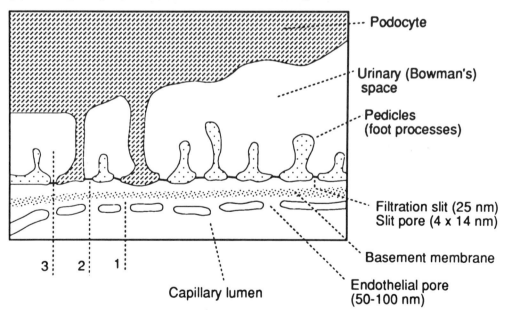

Figure 2–3. The filtration barrier. The numbers refer to size/mass of solute that can get through at that point: **1** (endothelial pores) permits the passage of red blood cells (50 to 100 nm diameter); **2** (basement membrane) permits passage of substances up to 8 nm or 500,000 MW; **3** (podocyte foot process) permits passage of substances up to the size of albumin (3.6 nm, 68,000 MW). × 70,000.

than 1000 daltons (effective radius about 2 nm) pass readily, whereas those over 60,000 daltons (effective radius greater than 4 nm) are essentially retained. Between these two limits there is a variable amount of filtration.

Retention of large proteins, particularly albumin, by the filtration barrier is critical to maintenance of plasma oncotic pressure and, hence, plasma volume.

Characteristics of Solutes that Influence Filtration. The shape, size, and flexibility of solute molecules influence filtration across the glomerular filtration barrier. Net electrical charge also plays an important role.

The importance of charge was discovered using dextrans. Dextrans are polysaccharides that can be produced in a wide range of molecular weights and charges. As seen in Figure 2–4, at any given effective molecular radius, the positively charged (anionic) dextrans pass through the glomerular filter more readily than do uncharged dextrans. Negatively charged (catatonic) dextrans are filtered even less readily than are uncharged dextrans. This selective filterability is explained by the presence of anionic sites in the capillary wall. Studies indicate that these polyanionic sites consist largely of heparin sulfate proteoglycans and sialoproteins, especially in the basal lamina. In other words, **the glomerular capillary wall, in addition to discriminating on the basis of size, also acts as an electrostatic barrier.**

Difference in Protein Composition Between Plasma and Glomerular Filtrate. **A solute that is partially bound to plasma proteins will have a lower concentration**

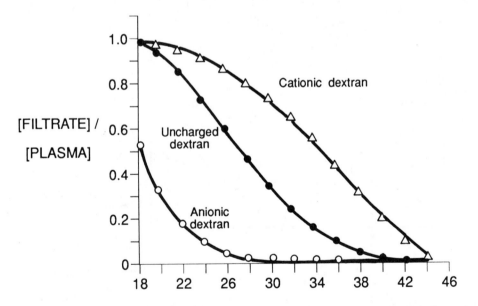

Figure 2–4. Filtrate/plasma ratios for uncharged, anionic, and cationic dextrans as a function of effective radius. (*Adapted from Bohrer MP, Baylis C, Humes HD, et al: Permselectivity of the glomerular capillary wall. Facilitated filtration of circulating polycations. J Clin Invest 1978; 61:72.*)

in Bowman's space because the protein-bound moiety is not filtered. The concentration of a filterable solute in Bowman's space equals the free, that is, the unbound, concentration in the plasma.

The Mesangium. Since the glomerular capillaries are embedded within the mesangium, only the capillary wall apposed to the visceral surface of Bowman's capsule provides filtration. Other parts of the capillary wall face inward to the mesangial core. The mesangium, in which the branching and anastomosing capillaries are embedded, is composed of mesangial cells and an extracellular matrix. The mesangial cells possess contractile properties and are stimulated directly by a variety of circulating hormones as well as renal nerves. Evidence now exists that contraction of the mesangium can control glomerular filtration through regulation of available filtration surface of the glomerular capillaries.

Determinants of Glomerular Filtration Rate

The critical factors that influence GFR include Starling forces, characteristics of the glomerular capillaries, and other physiologic factors.

Starling Forces. Movement of fluid across all capillary membranes, including the glomerular tuft, is determined by Starling filtration–reabsorption forces (Fig. 2–5). The three specific factors include (1) the transcapillary hydraulic pressure gradient, (2) the transcapillary oncotic pressure gradient, and (3) the glomerular capillary filtration coefficient.

Differences Between Glomerular Capillaries and Systemic Capillaries. There are several significant differences in fluid exchange across glomerular capillaries and across systemic capillaries.

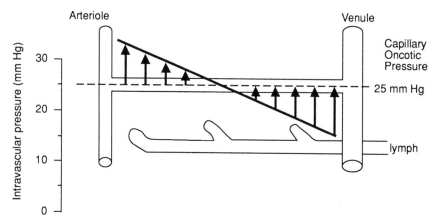

Figure 2–5. Diagram of fluid shifts along an average capillary (Starling force). Filtrate flow is depicted by vertical arrows.

High Constant Hydraulic Pressure. Hydraulic pressure in glomerular capillaries is higher and remains relatively constant, whereas it declines markedly along the length of systemic capillaries.

High Hydraulic Pressure in Bowman's Space. Hydraulic pressure in Bowman's space is greater than in systemic tissues.

Lower Permeability to Protein. The glomerular capillaries leak less protein than systemic capillaries. Thus, the oncotic pressure is near zero in Bowman's space. This also retards filtration.

As protein-free fluid is filtered along the length of the glomerular capillaries, the plasma protein concentration increases progressively. This produces a rise in the capillary oncotic pressure. The net filtration pressure declines in glomerular capillaries mainly because plasma oncotic pressure rises. This is in contrast to nonrenal capillaries, in which the decline in net filtration pressure is caused principally by a decrease in capillary hydraulic pressure. This increase in plasma protein concentration imposes constraints on the filtration process toward the end of the capillary bed.

High Filtration Coefficient. Physiologists define the filtration coefficient, K_f, as the product of the surface area available for filtration and the effective hydraulic permeability (amount of water that penetrates the membrane for each mm Hg of pressure). Both factors probably are involved when K_f changes in glomerular capillaries.

Fluid transport is much higher in glomerular than systemic capillaries. Measurements show that the filtration coefficient in glomerular capillaries is about 10 to 100 times larger than values reported for other capillaries.

Other Physiologic Factors

Vasoactive Agents. Vasodilators increase and vasoconstrictors decrease RBF. Glomerular permeability is altered in both cases in the opposite direction from RBF, resulting in a constant filtration rate.

Renal Nerves. GFR falls more than 50% following high-frequency stimulation of renal nerves. The fall in GFR is attributed to both a decrease in K_f and a decrease in plasma flow.

Tubuloglomerular Feedback. In addition to vasoactive substances and renal nerves, **GFR also is controlled by the rate of urine (tubular fluid) delivery to the macula densa cells in the early distal tubule.** This is termed **tubuloglomerular feedback.** High flow rates or increased sodium chloride cause a fall in GFR through increased preglomerular and postglomerular arteriolar resistances and a decline in K_f. This reflex mechanism prevents excessive fluid and electrolyte loss when proximal nephron reabsorption is impaired.

In summary, hormones, other vasoactive substances, tubuloglomerular feedback, and renal nerves affect glomerular filtration by modulating the vascular tone of glomerular arterioles and mesangium.

The Concept of Clearance and Its Measurement

The Clearance Concept. Several body organs (eg, lungs, liver, kidneys, skin) are involved in removing or clearing different substances from plasma by metabolism or excretion.

Figure 2–6 illustrates three examples of renal transport that help clarify the clearance concept. Substance **A** is cleared totally from blood by a process of filtration and secretion (eg, PAH). Substance **B** is filtered but neither secreted nor reabsorbed. Its clearance results totally from filtration (eg, inulin). Substance **C** is filtered at the same rate as **B**, but since it is totally reabsorbed, its clearance is 0 (eg, glucose). Some substances may undergo all three processes simultaneously.

Definition of Clearance. Clearance is defined as **the volume of plasma from which a substance is completely removed (cleared) per unit time.** This is an apparent and not an actual rate—rather, a little of the substance is removed

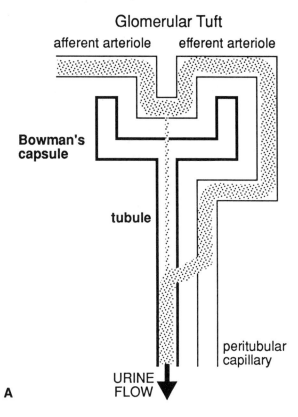

Glomerular Tuft

afferent arteriole   efferent arteriole

Bowman's capsule

tubule

peritubular capillary

URINE FLOW

A

Figure 2–6. Illustration of renal transport of three substances. Substance **A** is filtered and secreted. (continued.)

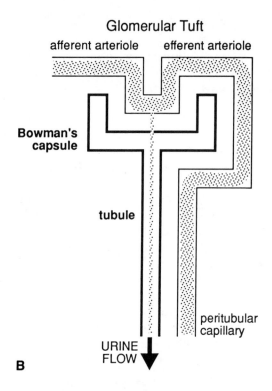

B

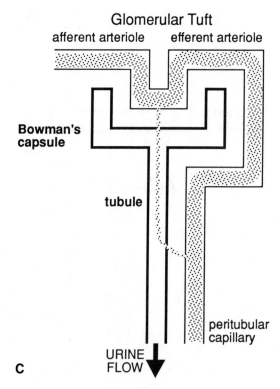

Figure 2–6 (continued). Renal
transport of three substances.
Substance **B** is only filtered.
Substance **C** is filtered and
reabsorbed.

C

continuously from each of the many milliliters of plasma perfusing an excretory organ.

The renal clearance of any substance is defined as the volume of plasma from which that substance is removed per unit time to supply the amount of the substance that is excreted in the urine in the same period of time.

Every substance in the plasma has a distinct renal clearance, usually expressed as milliliters per minute (mL/min). Most excreted substances are cleared by a combination of glomerular filtration and tubular secretion or reabsorption.

Clearance and GFR. **Glomerular filtration** is the initial process in the formation of urine. Substances removed (cleared) only by glomerular filtration can be used to measure GFR. During filtration, **serum passes through the glomerular capillary wall to produce a cell-free, low-protein fluid in Bowman's space.** This process is qualitatively the same as filtration across systemic capillaries to produce lymphatic fluid, but the two processes are quantitatively different. **The measurement of GFR involves a special application of the clearance concept.**

Inulin Clearance. Conceptually, if any substance in plasma (1) has the same concentration in both glomerular filtrate and plasma, (2) is not secreted, reabsorbed, synthesized, or degraded by the tubules, (3) is physiologically inert, and (4) can be measured, its renal clearance can be used to measure the GFR. Inulin, an uncharged fructose polymer weighing about 5000 daltons, meets all these criteria. The principal disadvantage of inulin is the need to infuse it intravenously to estimate GFR.

To illustrate calculation of GFR, consider the following hypothetical situation: Inulin is infused into a patient at a rate sufficient to maintain the plasma concentration at 4 mg/L. Urine collected over a 24-hour period has a volume of 2 L and an inulin concentration of 360 mg/L. Estimate the patient's GFR.

Inulin clearance (C_{in}) is used to estimate GFR.

$$C_{in} = GFR = \frac{[in]_u \times V}{[in]_p}$$

$$= \frac{360 \text{ mg/L} \times 2 \text{ L/day}}{4 \text{ mg/ml}}$$

$$= 180 \text{ L/day, or } 125 \text{ mL/min}$$

where [in] is inulin concentration
u is urine
p is plasma
V is volume

From the renal clearance equation, certain relationships of the plasma inulin concentration to both inulin clearance and inulin excretion rate can be examined. The results of several human studies are summarized in Figure 2–7. At a constant GFR, inulin excretion increases directly and linearly as a function of plasma inulin concentration (Fig. 2–7A). Inulin clearance is constant over a wide range of plasma inulin concentrations (Fig. 2–7B) and urine flow rates (Fig. 2–7C). These findings

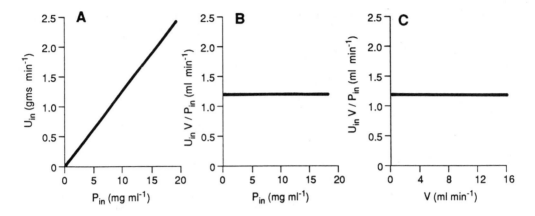

Figure 2–7. Relationship of **(A)** Inulin excretion rate to plasma concentration, **(B)** inulin clearance to plasma concentration, **(C)** inulin clearance to urine flow rate. U_{in} is urine inulin concentration. P_{in} is plasma inulin concentration, V is urine flow rate.

are consistent with a lack of inulin tubular transport. Such relationships are important because they provide the basis for analysis of tubular reabsorption and secretion by clearance methods. The range of inulin clearance in healthy men is 52 to 90 mL/min per square meter (m²) of body surface area, and it is 47 to 72 mL/min/ m² in women.

With a reliable method for measuring GFR, it is possible to evaluate whether a substance is reabsorbed or secreted by the renal tubules. For example, a substance that is not protein-bound and is freely filterable but has a lower rate of urinary excretion than inulin at the same plasma concentration has undergone net tubular reabsorption. A substance with a greater rate of excretion than that of inulin at the same plasma concentration obviously has been secreted by tubular cells.

Unfortunately, because of the need to infuse inulin intravenously, measuring GFR with inulin is inconvenient. Therefore, in clinical practice, an endogenous substance, creatinine, commonly is used to estimate GFR.

Creatinine Clearance (C_{cr}) and Plasma Creatinine [Cr]_p. Creatinine clearance or plasma creatinine alone usually is **used for clinical estimates of GFR.** Because of the importance of these tests, the rationale behind their use is described briefly.

ADVANTAGES. Creatinine is a metabolic waste product with a constant plasma concentration when renal function, dietary protein intake, and muscle mass are stable. Its assay is readily available in all clinical laboratories. The measurement of creatinine clearance requires only a single blood sample and a timed urine collection.

ASSUMPTIONS. The rationale behind use of creatinine clearance as a measure of GFR depends on four assumptions.

1. Constant creatinine production
2. Creatinine and inulin have similar renal handling
3. Accurate measurements
4. Accurate collections

PROBLEMS. Unfortunately, none of these four assumptions is strictly correct, but for clinical purposes, they are sufficiently accurate. Research studies usually require the greater precision of the inulin clearance test.

Overall, the chief virtue of creatinine clearance determination is its convenience. Use of creatinine clearance has a long clinical history for following renal function and for adjusting the dosage of some drugs dependent on renal excretion.

PLASMA CREATININE AS AN INDEX OF GFR. In practice, the plasma (or serum) creatinine concentration is widely used as an indicator of GFR. As the renal clearance equation indicates, **there is an inverse correlation between the plasma creatinine concentration and the creatinine clearance** (Fig. 2–8). Clinically, this information is useful in determining changes in GFR through single measurements of plasma creatinine concentration. The major advantages of this estimate of C_{cr} are that it is rapid and convenient and that it does not require a timed urine collection.

Example. A patient with an initial plasma creatinine of 1 mg/dL (10 mg/L) is later found to have slowly progressive renal failure with a plasma creatinine concentration of 2 mg/dL. If we assume steady state conditions (production =

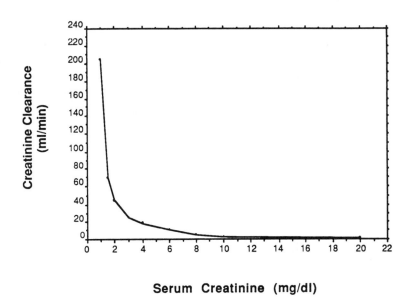

Serum Creatinine (mg/dl)

Figure 2–8. Inverse relationship between the plasma creatinine and the creatinine clearance.

urinary excretion + metabolism), it is clear that the GFR is one half of the previous value, or 90 L/day. (if we assume a previous normal GFR of 180 L/day).

$$\text{Initial steady state}$$
$$\text{Filtered creatinine} = 10 \text{ mg/L} \times 180 \text{ L/day}$$
$$= 1800 \text{ mg/day}$$
$$\text{New steady state}$$
$$\text{Filtered creatinine} = 20 \text{ mg/L} \times 90 \text{ L/day}$$
$$= 1800 \text{ mg/day}$$

From Figure 2–8, creatinine clearance has decreased from 120 mL/min to 60 mL/min. (This value also can be calculated from 90 L/day.)

There are **limitations of plasma creatinine as a measure of GFR.** With increasing renal failure, the precise relationship between the plasma creatinine concentration and GFR fails because creatinine production falls (loss of muscle mass), gut bacterial metabolism increases (due to catalytic enzyme enhancement), and substantial tubular secretion of creatinine develops. Therefore, plasma creatinine fails to rise proportionate to the fall in GFR. However, the relationship is still good enough to serve as a convenient tool for following patients with progressive renal failure.

Urea Clearance and Blood Urea Nitrogen (BUN). The renal clearance of urea historically was one of the first estimates of GFR. **Because urea is freely filtered by the glomeruli, the BUN varies inversely with GFR** in a manner analogous to the serum creatinine (Fig. 2–9). However, **we now recognize that urea clearance and BUN are poor measures of renal function.**

UREA CLEARANCE DEPENDS ON URINE FLOW RATE. When compared with inulin or creatinine renal clearances, the urea clearance is lower, and it depends on the urine flow rate (Fig. 2–9). It is now clear that urea undergoes a complex intrarenal recycling process that is related to circulating antidiuretic hormone (ADH or vasopressin) concentration and water reabsorption in the cortical and medullary collecting ducts. Thus, urea clearance is a poor estimate of GFR.

LIMITATIONS OF BUN AS INDEX OF RENAL FUNCTION. Because so many other factors (eg, catabolism, liver function, diet) affect the BUN, it is not a good index of renal function.

CLINICAL USE OF BUN CONCENTRATION. Although it reflects GFR poorly, the BUN does provide useful clinical information in a number of situations: (1) If the dietary protein intake is about 1 g/kg/day, **a BUN concentration between 10 and 15 mg/dL will likely be associated with a normal GFR, and** (2) A BUN concentration less **than 10 mg/dL usually reflects low dietary protein intake, states of overhydration (increased urea distribution volume), or severe liver disease.**

BUN/CREATININE RATIO. Although the absolute BUN concentration is not an accurate estimate of the GFR, **the ratio of the BUN and serum creatinine concentrations**

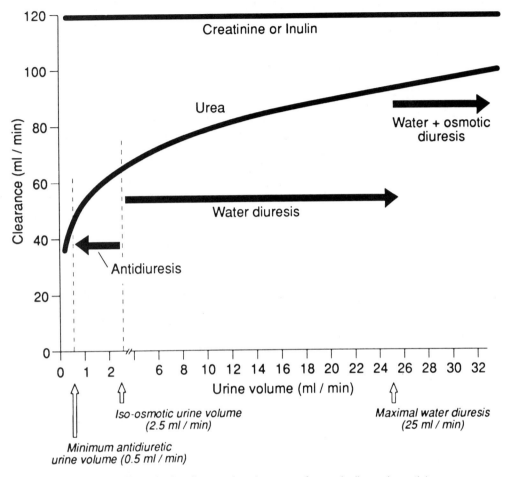

Figure 2–9. The effect of urine flow on the clearance of urea, inulin, and creatinine.

(BUN/creatinine) is useful for determining the cause of a diminished GFR or suggesting certain nonrenal events.

1. A ratio **greater than 15:1 indicates either prerenal causes of a reduced GFR (ECF volume depletion, heart failure) or postrenal obstruction (stones, tumors) of urine flow (in the absence of excess protein intake, gastrointestinal bleeding, or increased catabolism).** Each cause is associated with low tubular urine flow and a high degree of intrarenal urea reabsorption.
2. **A BUN/creatinine ratio of 15:1** in a patient with renal insufficiency is consistent with a primary renal disorder.
3. **In advanced renal failure, the BUN/creatinine ratio is approximately 15:1 because the clearance of both creatinine and urea are comparably impaired. Lower ratios are usually associated with low dietary protein intake or hepatic insufficiency (with decreased urea production).**

REGULATION OF RENAL BLOOD FLOW AND GLOMERULAR FILTRATION RATE

Importance of Maintaining Constant RBF and GFR

Changes in RBF have the potential to significantly alter GFR. The resulting **changes in GFR would cause large changes in water and salt excretion.** Thus, it is important for the body to prevent large fluctuations in GFR. To maintain a constant internal environment, the kidneys have an intrinsic ability to maintain the RBF and GFR nearly constant, despite wide fluctuations in arterial pressure.

Concept of Renal Autoregulation

Use of animal models has clarified the concept of renal autoregulation. When the renal arterial pressure in a denervated, blood-perfused dog kidney was increased from 10 to 80 mm Hg, both RBF and GFR increased linearly (Fig. 2–10). Further increases in blood pressure beyond 80 mm Hg led to no change in either GFR or RBF until renal arterial pressure reached 180 mm Hg. Increasing renal arterial pressure above 180 mm Hg caused an increase in RBF. However, there was no change in GFR. This experiment illustrates that RBF and GFR are maintained at constant levels over a wide (physiologic) range of systemic blood pressures. **The ability of the kidney to maintain GFR and RBF constant despite wide fluctuations in systemic arterial pressure is called autoregulation.**

Mechanisms of Renal Autoregulation

Renal autoregulation of RBF and GFR is accomplished by a combination of intrinsic and extrinsic mechanisms.

Intrinsic Mechanisms. The intrinsic mechanisms of autoregulation occur **within the kidney.** There are three possible intrinsic mechanisms responsible for autoregulation of renal blood flow: (1) myogenic feedback, (2) tubuloglomerular feedback, and (3) the renin–angiotensin–prostaglandin system.

Myogenic Mechanism. The myogenic theory proposes that the arteriolar muscular tone is the key to renal autoregulation. As seen in Figure 2–10, RBF increases linearly as systemic blood pressure rises to 80 mm Hg. During this phase, renal vascular resistance remains constant.

At systemic blood pressures in the range of 80 to 180 mm Hg, there is no change in RBF. Thus, over this wide range of systemic blood pressures, the renal arterial resistance (R) must increase to maintain constant RBF. This increase in renal arteriolar resistance (with increase in pressure) is believed to reflect an increase in afferent arteriolar tone as arterial pressure increases.

Tubuloglomerular Feedback. The ascending limb of the loop of Henle returns to pass by the glomerulus at the juxtaglomerular apparatus (JGA). The **macula densa cells sense the sodium concentration in the tubule and adjust the GFR by caus-**

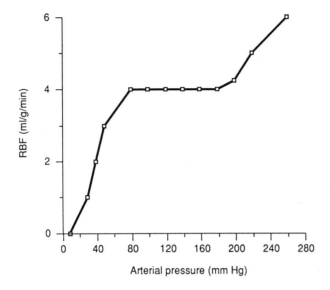

Figure 2–10. Autoregulation of renal blood flow (RBF) in the dog.

ing the afferent arteriole to constrict or relax. If sodium is high, the afferent arteriole constricts; if it is low, the afferent arteriole dilates.

In summary, the tubuloglomerular feedback mechanism has the capacity to exert a negative feedback control on arteriolar inflow and GFR.

Renin–angiotensin System. The renin–angiotensin system is the third intrarenal mechanism mediating autoregulation. The renin–angiotensin system is stimulated when the renal perfusion pressure falls below the lower limit of normal systemic pressure. Renin release from the JGA leads to conversion of angiotensin I to angiotensin II within the kidney. Angiotensin II is a powerful vasoconstrictor that increases efferent arteriolar tone, thereby maintaining GFR. All three intrinsic mechanisms may function in complementary fashion to ensure autoregulation.

Extrinsic Mechanisms. Systemic factors also regulate RBF and GFR. These extrinsic mechanisms for renal autoregulation are of two types: neural and humoral. Several factors involved are noted in Table 2–1. The multiple levels of controls serving to assure autoregulation emphasize the importance of maintaining a constant RBF and GFR.

MEASUREMENT OF RENAL BLOOD FLOW

Determination of PAH clearance is one of the most common methods for measuring RBF. At low serum concentrations (< 10mg/dL), PAH is removed completely from the blood during a single passage through the kidney. Since clearance of any

TABLE 2–1. FACTORS AFFECTING RENAL BLOOD FLOW

Model	Renal Blood Flow	Renal Resistance
Dopamine	▲	▼
Hydralazine	▲	▼
Epinephrine[a]	▼	▲
Saline diuresis	▲	▼
Furosemide	▲	▼
Norepinephrine[a]	▼	▲
Angiotensin	▼	▲

[a]Naturally occurring hormones.
▼Decreased.
▲Increased.

substance is defined as the volume of plasma from which that substance is re-moved in a given time, clearance of PAH equals the renal plasma flow at low concentrations of PAH. If PAH concentration is high, not all of the PAH will be cleared from the plasma during a single passage through the kidney. In this situation, PAH clearance will be significantly less than the renal plasma flow.

SAMPLE ANSWERS TO STUDY QUESTIONS

1. a. How much plasma flows through normal adult kidneys in 1 day?

660 mL/min $\times$ 1440 min/day = 940.4 L/day

b. Why is such a large plasma volume needed by the kidneys?

This large plasma volume is needed to provide sufficiently large glomerular filtration and to maintain the internal environment.

2. a. Define the filtration fraction (FF).

FF is the proportion of plasma flow that is filtered at the glomeruli.
FF = GFR/RPF
Normal FF = $\dfrac{130 \text{ mL/min}}{660 \text{ mL/min}}$ = 0.2

b. If the FF is 30% and renal plasma flow (RPF) is 660 mL/min, is the glomerular filtration rate (GFR) normal, subnormal or higher than normal?

Since
FF = GFR/RPF, GFR = FF X RPF.
In this case, GFR = 660 $\times$ 0.3 = 198. This is higher than normal.

3. a. Name the major sites of renal resistance.

Afferent arteriole, efferent arteriole, and venules.

b. What is the significance of afferent and efferent arteriolar pressure?

Interplay of the afferent and efferent arteriolar pressures maintains a constant intraglomerular pressure and, consequently, a constant GFR.

4. a. What is autoregulation, and why is it important?

Renal autoregulation is the intrinsic ability of the kidney to maintain RBF and GFR constant despite physiologic fluctuations in systemic arterial pressure.

b. In what pressure range is autoregulation operative?

A range of 80 to 180 mm Hg.

5.a. What happens to GFR if afferent arteriolar resistance increases?

The intraglomerular pressure and, consequently, the GFR declines if other forces are unchanged.

b. What happens if efferent arteriolar resistance increases?

If other forces are unchanged, the GFR increases.

6. If the para-aminohippurate (PAH) concentration in blood is high (> 15 mg/ dL), would PAH clearance be equal to, less than, or greater than renal plasma flow (RPF)?

PAH clearance would be less than RPF. If all PAH is cleared from the plasma in a single pass through the kidney, RPF = PAH clearance. However, at high PAH concentrations, some PAH is left in the plasma. This means that the volume of plasma that is cleared of PAH (PAH clearance) would be less than the RPF.

7. From the data given, calculate the renal clearance of (a) inulin, (b) urea, and (c) para-aminohippurate (PAH).

$$[\text{inulin}]_u = 100 \text{ mg/dL}$$
$$[\text{inulin}]_p = 1 \text{ mg/dL}$$
$$[\text{urea}]_u = 220 \text{ mmol/L}$$
$$[\text{urea}]_p = 5 \text{ mmol/L}$$
$$[\text{PAH}]_u = 1000 \text{ mg/dL}$$
$$[\text{PAH}]_p = 2 \text{ mg/dL}$$

a. Inulin clearance

$$C_{in} = GFR = \frac{[inulin]_u \times V}{[inulin]_p}$$

$$= \frac{100 \text{ mg/dl} \times 1.4 \text{ L/day}}{1 \text{ mg/dL}}$$

$$= 140 \text{ L/day or 100 mL/min}$$

b. Urea clearance

$$C_{urea} = \frac{[urea]_u \times V}{[urea]_p}$$

$$= \frac{220 \text{ mmol/L} \times 1.4 \text{ L/day}}{5 \text{ mmol/L}}$$

$$= 61.6 \text{ L/day or 44 mL/min}$$

c. PAH clearance

$$C_{PAH} = \frac{[PAH]_u \times V}{[PAH]_p}$$

$$= \frac{1000 \text{ mg/dL} \times 1.4 \text{ L/day}}{2 \text{ mg/dL}}$$

$$= 700 \text{ L/day or 406 mL/min}$$

Tubular Transport

INTRODUCTION

This chapter considers how urine is formed by the kidney and how substances are removed, or cleared, from the blood. Urine is produced by three mechanisms (Fig. 3–1): (1) glomerular filtration, (2) tubular reabsorption, and (3) tubular secretion. Tubular reabsorption and tubular secretion are discussed in this chapter.

STUDY QUESTIONS

1. Renal excretion of substance **A** is less than that of inulin despite similar plasma concentrations. Give three possible explanations.
2. Substance **B** is filtered, reabsorbed, and secreted. How would you design a system for increasing the renal excretion of this substance?
3. A 55 year-old man with benign prostatic hyperplasia (BPH) was found on initial examination to weigh 72 kg and to have a serum creatinine of 1.2 mg/dL and a creatinine clearance (C_{cr}) of 60 mL/min. Assuming the data to be accurate, why is the serum creatinine concentration in the normal range whereas the C_{cr} appears low?
4. The patient in Question 2 was seen 5 years later for symptoms of bladder outlet

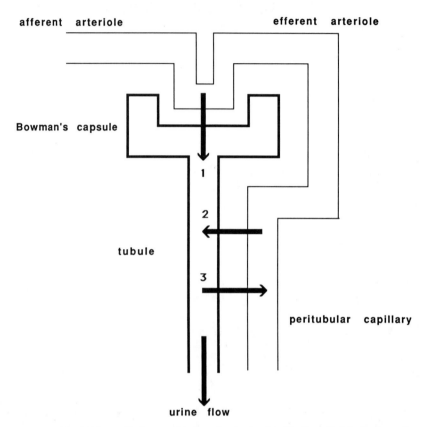

Figure 3–1. Mechanism of urine production: **1**, glomerular filtration, **2**, tubular secretion, **3**, tubular reabsorption.

obstruction. At this time, his weight was still 72 kg, but his serum creatinine was 3.6 mg/dL. You can estimate his current C_{cr} if you make certain assumptions. What must you assume, and what is your estimate of C_{cr}?

5. You are asked to see a patient who was hospitalized recently for severe gastro-enteritis associated with fluid and electrolyte disturbances. The serum creatinine and BUN concentrations are 2 mg/dL and 45 mg/dL, respectively. Discuss possible reasons for these values.

TUBULAR TRANSPORT

Functional Divisions of the Renal Tubule

Based on major functional characteristics, the renal tubule can be divided into **four segments** (Table 3–1). Although the analogy is imperfect, the renal tubule has

TABLE 3–1. FUNCTIONAL DIVISIONS OF THE RENAL TUBULE

Anatomic Segment	Physiologic Function
Proximal tubule	Reabsorption
Loop of Henle	Concentration and dilution
Distal convoluted tubule	Final adjustments
Collecting tubule	Final adjustments

similarities to the gut. Proximal segments (proximal convoluted tubules, small intestines) are principally involved in reabsorption of fluid and solutes with secretion of some metabolites, whereas the distal segments (collecting tubules, colon) exert a final adjustment to the excretion of solutes and fluid. The loop of Henle and associated vasa recta are involved in diluting and concentrating the urine, a unique function of the kidney without an intestinal counterpart.

Methods for Measuring Tubular Functions

Renal tubular functions may be measured using either direct or indirect methods.

Direct methods include invasive techniques to measure concentration of various solutes, pH, or electrical voltage at different points along the renal tubule. The two types of direct methods involve **micropuncture** and **microperfusion** studies. The direct methods are chiefly used for **experimental studies** in animals.

Indirect methods use **noninvasive** techniques for measuring renal tubular function. The major indirect method for evaluating tubular function is the **renal clearance technique.** This is the only method that is applicable to **clinical situations.**

Types of Tubular Transport

Transfer of substances across the renal tubule occurs by either passive mechanisms or active mechanisms (Fig. 3–2).

I. **Passive Transport.** Passive mechanisms have three distinguishing **characteristics.**
   A. **Following gradients.** In passive transport, a substance diffuses along an electric or chemical gradient.
   B. **Energy is not directly required** but may be necessary to establish the initial gradient.
   C. **Both transcellular and extracellular routes.** The fraction of tubular diffusion that occurs through transcellular routes (across both apical and basolateral membranes) versus that which bypasses the cell through paracellular spaces (Fig. 3–2) is controversial. If the junctional complexes are highly permeable, as in the proximal tubule, any electrochemical gradient is dissipated quickly by paracellular solute and water transport. Such permeability allows large amounts of water and solutes to be reabsorbed with a minimum of energy. Where it is critical to develop large

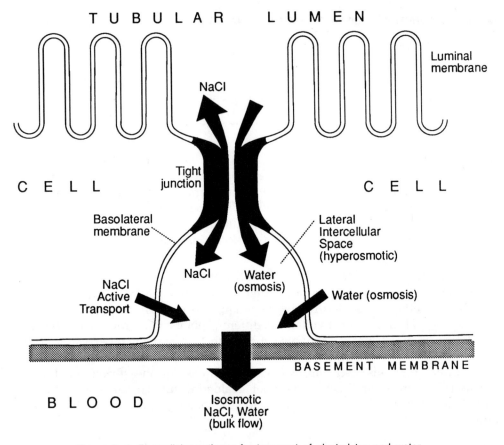

Figure 3–2. Paracellular pathway for transport of electrolytes and water.

concentration gradients, junctional complexes have low permeabilities, as in the distal nephron.

II. **Active transport.** There are three distinguishing characteristics of active transport processes.

    A. **Against gradients.** With active transport, a substance moves against a chemical or electric gradient.

    B. **Energy required.** Direct expenditure of energy is necessary for movement of substances against such electrochemical gradients.

    C. **Transcellular pathways.** In contrast to passive transport, active transport uses only transcellular pathways.

    D. Examples of active transport.

        i. **Endocytosis.** Although not often considered in this context, endocytosis is a specific form of active transport involving **macromolecules.** This process involves binding of a substance to the plasma membrane and invagination of that section of the membrane until it is completely pinched off and exists as an intracellular, plasma membrane-lined vesicle.

    ii. **Other molecules.** The classic examples of active renal tubular reabsorption and secretion are **D-glucose** (dextrose) and **PAH** respectively. Figure 3–3 shows the typical renal excretion curves for these substances in comparison with inulin.

E. **Limitations to active transport.** Theoretically, any active process has quantitative limits. Active renal transport processes fall into two general categories, those associated with a **transport maximum (T_m)** and those showing a limitation in the gradient developed between the peritubular blood and tubular lumen.

    i. **T_m-limited active transport.** Substances showing T_m-limited characteristics are **glucose, amino acids, phosphate, sulfate, and organic acids. Their transport mechanisms can handle only a certain quantity of the substance (eg, approximately 300 mg/min for glucose).**

    ii. **Gradient-limited active transport.** The gradient-limited pattern is seen in the transport of **sodium, potassium, and hydrogen ions.** These processes **can handle very large quantities but cannot overcome large gradients.**

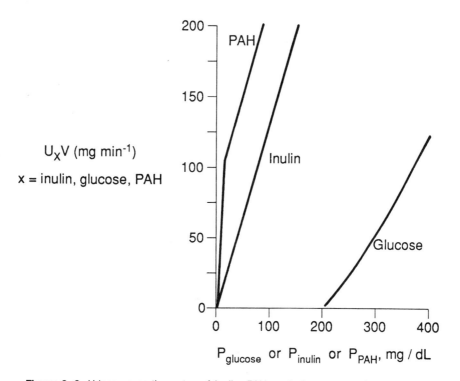

Figure 3–3. Urinary excretion rates of inulin, PAH, and glucose as a function of their plasma levels.

Tubular Reabsorption

Glucose

Normal Reabsorption. The reabsorptive mechanism for glucose is an example of **an active T_m-limited tubular transport system. With normal plasma glucose concentrations (90 to 100 mg/dL) and GFR (70 mL/min/m²), glucose is not found in the urine.** Since glucose is filtered freely at the glomerulus, it must be completely reabsorbed. Micropuncture studies show that glucose recovery has occurred by the end of the proximal tubule. Indeed, approximately halfway along the proximal tubule, the concentration of glucose is zero, indicating that the nephron possesses considerable reserve for recovering filtered glucose. The rest of the nephron is impermeable to glucose.

Glucosuria with Hyperglycemia. Although glucose is not normally found in urine, **it is possible to produce glucosuria in normal people by administering large quantities of glucose intravenously, producing hyperglycemia and increasing the**

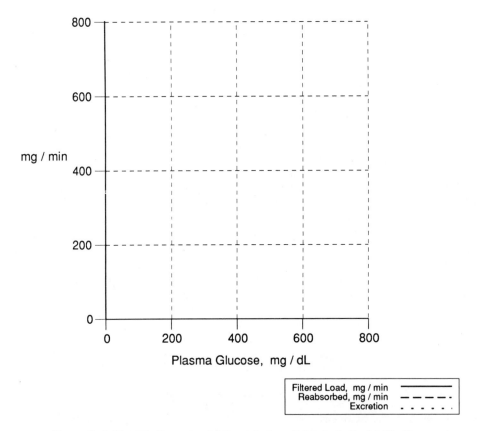

Figure 3–4. Use this figure to plot the data from Table 3–2. Depict filtration, reabsorption, and excretion as a function of plasma level.

filtered glucose load above the reabsorptive capacity (T_m) (Fig. 3–4, Table 3–2).

Even after the plasma glucose concentration has been doubled, the urine is still free of glucose, indicating that maximal tubular transport capacity for reabsorbing glucose has not yet been reached. As the plasma glucose and the filtered load continue to rise, glucose finally appears in the urine. From this point on, any further increase in plasma glucose is accompanied by a proportional increase in excreted glucose, because the T_m, **which equals 216 mg/min/m²**, has now been reached. **The tubules are now reabsorbing all the glucose they can, and any amount filtered in excess of this quantity cannot be reabsorbed and, therefore, appears in the urine.** This is precisely **what occurs in the patient with diabetes mellitus when the plasma concentration of glucose is greatly elevated. There is nothing wrong with the tubular transport mechanisms for glucose. The kidneys simply are unable to reabsorb the large filtered load.**

Renal Glycosuria. **If the plasma glucose concentration is normal and glucose appears in the urine, reabsorption has somehow failed.** This relationship is demonstrated **experimentally** following treatment with a **specific inhibitor of glucose transport, phlorhizin.** In this situation, massive glycosuria occurs, and the renal clearance of glucose equals the GFR, although no other evidence of renal dysfunction is present. The defect is transient and disappears once phlorhizin is excreted.

Clinically, a number of **congenital disorders** associated with renal glycosuria resemble the defect produced by phlorhizin. In some of these disorders, the reabsorptive mechanism may fail only for glucose. More **often, there are other associated proximal tubule defects.**

Amino Acids. The concentration of amino acids in plasma ranges from 2.5 to 3.5 mmol/L and is determined by a dynamic balance among intestinal absorption of amino acids, protein catabolism into urea and ammonia, and cellular synthesis of protein. One **major task of the kidney is recovery of the large amounts of amino acids that are filtered** by the glomeruli each day. With normal plasma levels, little or no amino acids are found in the urine. Thus, the **renal clearance is zero.**

As the plasma concentration is raised by infusing amino acids intravenously, amino acid excretion occurs when the filtered load exceeds a threshold value.

TABLE 3–2. EXPERIMENTAL DATA OBTAINED FOR CALCULATION OF GLUCOSE T_m

Time (min)	GFR (mL/min)	Plasma Glucose ($G[_p]$) (mg/mL)	Filtered Glucose (GFR × $G[_p]$) (mg/min)	Excreted Glucose ($[G]_{UV}$) (mg/min)	Reabsorbed Glucose (filtered-excreted) (mg/min)
0	125	1.0	125	0	125
		Begin Glucose Infusion			
26–140	125	2.0	250	0	250
110–110	125	4.0	500	125	370
130–140	125	5.0	625	250	375
160–170	125	6.0	750	375	375

These properties suggest that amino acids are absorbed by **an active transport mechanism with a T_m-limited capacity.**

Proteins. Although the glomerular filtration barrier is relatively impermeable to plasma proteins, **small amounts do escape into the filtrate.** The protein concentration in the filtrate has been estimated to be 200 mg/L and is osmotically trivial compared to the 70 g/L in plasma. In terms of potential protein loss through the kidney, however, this concentration of protein in the glomerular filtrate is significant considering the high GFR.

$$\text{Total filtered protein} = \text{GFR} \times \text{filtered concentration of protein}$$
$$= 180 \text{ L/day} \times 200 \text{ mg/L}$$
$$= 36 \text{ g/day}$$

The virtual absence of protein in the final urine (less than 150 mg/day) despite glomerular filtration of 30 to 40 g/day is evidence of tubular resorption.

Tubular Secretion

In addition to glomerular filtration, tubular secretion represents a pathway into the tubular lumen. Tubular secretion is the **processes of transport from the peritubular blood into the lumen.** This starts with simple diffusion into the interstitial space and hence into the lumen via the tight junction or across the basolateral and luminal membranes by active or passive processes.

Important electrolytes demonstrating net tubular secretion include **hydrogen and potassium ions.** Secretory mechanisms for **organic acids** (anions) **and bases** (cations) also exist. Many exogenous substances (**foods, drugs**) also are secreted by routes that, like reabsorptive processes, demonstrate specificity, saturability, and competition.

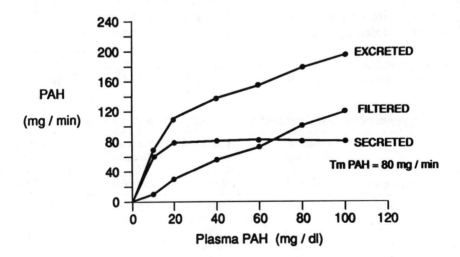

Figure 3–5. Filtration, secretion, and excretion of PAH as a function of its plasma level.

The best known and studied of these compounds is the organic acid, PAH, which is secreted by a T_m-limited mechanism. The excretion curve differs from that of a purely filtered substance (inulin) or a reabsorbed substance (glucose). Excretion of PAH always is greater than either its filtration or secretion curves (Fig. 3–5). When T_m is reached, the excretion rate differs from the filtration rate by a constant amount (the T_m), and the excretion and filtration rates are parallel.

Bidirectional Tubular Transport

Although most organic acids are secreted by the kidney, a number of naturally occurring organic anions undergo both secretion and reabsorption, often by the same nephron segment. Most clinically relevant in this context is **uric acid**, the major end product of purine catabolism.

SAMPLE ANSWERS TO STUDY QUESTIONS

1. **Renal excretion of substance A is less than that of inulin despite similar plasma concentrations. Give three possible explanations.**

   Substance **A** may be
   (a) Too large (> 20,000 daltons) to be filtered by the glomeruli, (b) Bound to plasma macromolecules, or (c) Reabsorbed by the tubules once it is filtered.

2. **Substance B is filtered, reabsorbed, and secreted. How would you design a system for increasing the renal excretion of this substance?**

   There are three possibilities (either alone or in combination).
   (a) Increase filtered substance **B** by increasing either GFR or plasma concentration of substance **B**, (b) Inhibit tubular reabsorption of substance **B**, or (c) Enhance tubular secretion of substance **B**.

3. **A 55-year-old man with benign prostatic hyperplasia (BPH) was found on initial examination to weigh 72 kg and to have a serum creatinine of 1.2 mg/dL and a creatinine clearance (C_{cr}) of 60 mL/min. Assuming the data to be accurate, why is the serum creatinine concentration in the normal range whereas the C_{cr} appears low?**

   The serum creatinine concentration is determined by the balance between production (metabolized from muscle creatine phosphate) and excretion (glomerular filtration and tubular secretion). A decrease in the serum creatinine concentration could result from a decrease in production (muscle atrophy) or an increase in GFR. With normal aging, muscle mass declines. Coincidentally, renal function falls in a parallel fashion from nephrosclerosis. Thus, the serum creatinine concentration remains constant. Presumably, in this individual, a rise in serum creatinine has not occurred because decreased production has paralleled decreased excretion.

4. **The patient in Question 2 was seen 5 years later for symptoms of bladder outlet obstruction. At this time, his weight was still 72 kg, but his serum creatinine was 3.6 mg/dL. You can estimate his current C_{cr} if you make certain assumptions. What must you assume, and what is your estimate of C_{cr}?**

You must assume
(a) The constant weight reflects no change in muscle mass
(b) Creatinine degradation by the gut is unchanged
(c) Production and elimination rates are constant
The three-fold rise in serum creatinine concentration (1.2 mg/dL to 3.6 mg/dL) is caused by a fall in C_{cr} to one third of the prior value, or 20 mL/min.

5. **You are asked to see a patient who was hospitalized recently for severe gastroenteritis associated with fluid and electrolyte disturbances. The serum creatinine and BUN concentrations are 2 mg/dL and 45 mg/dL, respectively. Discuss possible reasons for these values.**

The rise in serum creatinine and BUN indicates either an increase in creatinine and urea production or a decrease in elimination rates. The clinical history suggests extracellular fluid (ECF) volume depletion from gastrointestinal losses due to gastroenteritis. ECF volume depletion could reduce renal blood flow and urine flow rates. The former would decrease both creatinine and urea renal clearances, but the latter would have an additional effect of reducing urea renal clearance. Although the history does not suggest gastrointestinal bleeding, if this were present, the blood (protein) in the gut could increase the urea production rate. Either or both of these factors would explain the increase in serum concentrations and the high serum BUN/creatinine ratio.

Renal Handling of Sodium

INTRODUCTION

This chapter considers the various established mechanisms that affect renal control of sodium and water balance in health. Sodium is the principal cation in the extracellular fluid (ECF). Because sodium and an attendant anion are the major regulators of extracellular osmolarity, water balance and distribution are regulated largely by the sodium balance.

STUDY QUESTIONS

1. Write the equation relating filtration, reabsorption, and excretion of sodium.
2. For each 150 mmol of sodium chloride or sodium bicarbonate reabsorbed by the proximal tubule, how much water is reabsorbed?

3. Where is the site of osmotic equilibration between solutes and water in the proximal tubule?
4. How does mannitol, an osmotic diuretic, inhibit the recovery of salt and water in the proximal tubule?
5. Compare salt and water transport in the proximal tubule with that in the thick ascending limb and the collecting duct.
6. Calculate the fractional sodium excretion (percent of the filtered sodium excreted) from the following data.
   [sodium]$_p$ = 144 mmol/L
   [sodium]$_u$ = 200 mmol/L
   urine flow = 36 ml/30 min
      Cl$_{inulin}$ = 120 mL/min
7. A normal adult reduces daily sodium ingestion from 150 to 10 mmol. Describe the sequential daily changes in
   a. Body weight
   b. ECF volume
   c. Serum sodium concentration
   d. Daily urinary sodium excretion
8. Describe the same changes listed in Question 7 in a patient with renal failure (Cl$_{cr}$ = 10 mL/min) whose dietary sodium is reduced from 150 to 10 mmol/day.

INTRARENAL REGULATION OF SODIUM SALTS

The kidneys of the average adult filter about 180 L of water and 25,000 mmol of sodium salts daily. However, only **about 1% of the filtered amount is excreted in the urine. The rest is reabsorbed by the tubular cells.** Indeed, most renal energy is spent in reabsorbing sodium.

The mechanisms for reabsorption vary somewhat in different segments of the renal tubule, but two generalizations can be made that apply to all tubular segments except the loop of Henle.

1. Sodium reabsorption is an active process
2. Chloride and water reabsorption are passive and linked to the active transport of sodium

In the descending limb of the loop of Henle, water transport occurs without much solute movement. In the ascending limb, chloride transport is an active process, sodium movement is passive, and water diffusion does not occur. These unique characteristics of the loop of Henle are important in the production of a dilute or concentrated urine and are described in more detail in Chapter 5.

Proximal Convoluted Tubule

Proportional Reabsorption of Sodium and Water. Normally, 60 to 70% of filtered salt and water is reabsorbed in the proximal convoluted tubule (PCT). This reabsorption occurs without significant change in the tubular fluid sodium concen-

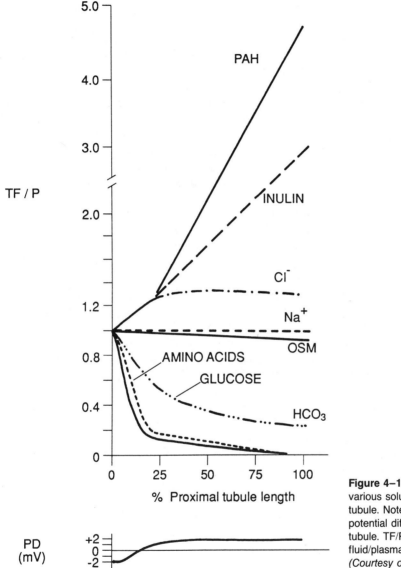

TF / P

PAH

INULIN

Cl⁻

Na⁺

OSM

AMINO ACIDS

GLUCOSE

HCO_3

% Proximal tubule length

PD
(mV)

Figure 4–1. Reabsorption of various solute along the proximal tubule. Note changes in the potential difference along the tubule. TF/P is the tubular fluid/plasma concentration ratio. *(Courtesy of F.C. Rector, Jr.)*

tration or osmolarity (Fig. 4–1). This indicates that **water and sodium are reab-sorbed at proportional rates.**

If the sodium concentration throughout the PCT is constant, what is the evidence that sodium reabsorption is an active process? Perhaps the best evidence comes from microperfusion studies. When sodium was replaced in the perfusate and bath by lithium or choline, fluid absorption ceased.

Sodium Reabsorption. Approximately 75% of reabsorbed sodium is accompanied by chloride, whereas the remaining 25% is transported with bicarbonate to maintain electrical neutrality.

Two thirds of the reabsorbed sodium is transported actively by three major mechanisms: unidirectional, $Na^+–H^+$ exchange, and Cl^--driven Na^+ exchange (Fig. 4–2). The remaining one third occurs by passive flow.

Unidirectional Transport of Sodium. This involves two steps, one active and one passive. The active step occurs at the basolateral borders of the tubular cells and requires energy from ATP for the enzymatic action of Na–K-ATPase at the cell membrane. This reaction extrudes sodium from the cell into peritubular fluid, producing a fall in the intracellular concentration of sodium. Since the intracellular sodium concentration is lower than that in both the luminal and peritubular fluid, a chemical gradient is created that moves sodium passively into the cell, mainly across the luminal border. In the early PCT, sodium movement is coupled with amino acid and glucose transport, and a small electrical potential is created. This potential difference (PD) is never large because of the high permeability of the PCT to chloride.

$Na^+–H^+$ Exchange. Sodium reabsorption from tubular fluid also occurs by exchange with intracellular hydrogen ions. **This is a countertransport system, where the movement of a substance in one direction provides the energy for the coupled movement of a second substance in the opposite direction.** Because of the fate of the H^+ secreted (Fig. 4–2B), the reabsorbed sodium produces transcellular transport of both chloride and bicarbonate.

Cl^--driven Exchange. Because of H^+ secretion, the luminal concentration of bicarbonate (about 8 mmol/L) falls (Fig. 4–2C), leaving a high concentration (about 132 mmol/L) of chloride. Since the peritubular concentration of these ions is similar to that in plasma, an ion concentration difference is produced. Since chloride is the more permeable ion, a lumen-positive transepithelial PD occurs that serves to retard Cl^- and favor Na^+ movement.

Passive Flow. Diffusive sodium chloride reabsorption occurs through paracellular routes because a favorable electrochemical gradient exists. Luminal chloride concentration is higher than the blood chloride concentration, and the lumen-positive electrical gradient drives sodium reabsorption.

Water Reabsorption. The presence of a paracellular pathway helps to explain water reabsorption in the PCT without a significant osmotic gradient across the cells. A possible sequence may be as follows. Sodium salts passively enter tubule cells across the luminal membrane and are extruded actively into the lateral intercellular space. Initially, salt concentration in the lateral spaces increases slightly relative to the luminal water movement into the lateral space by osmotic flow across both the cell and tight junction. The lateral space has a low compliance, and the influx of fluid produces an increase in hydraulic pressure in the lateral

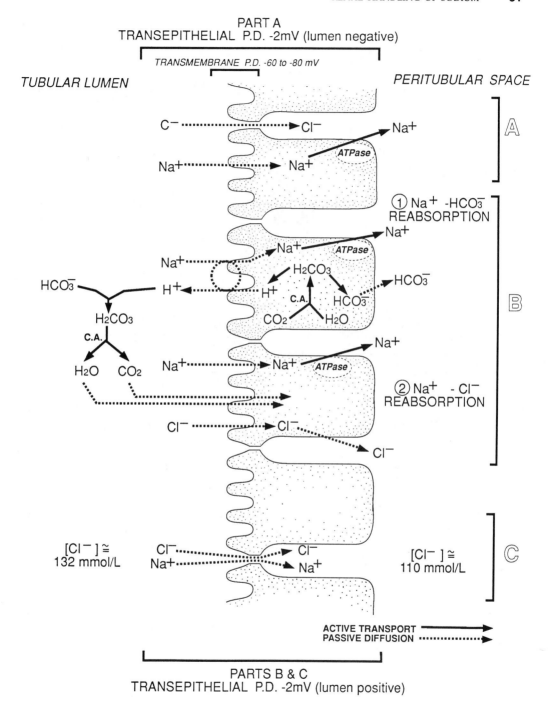

Figure 4–2. Mechanisms for active sodium reabsorption in the proximal tubule. **A.** Unidirectional transport of Na^+. **B.** Na^+–H^+ exchange. **C.** Cl^--driven exchange. *(From West JB, ed: Best and Taylor's Physiological Basis of Medical Practice, 11th ed. Baltimore: Williams and Wilkins, 1985.)*

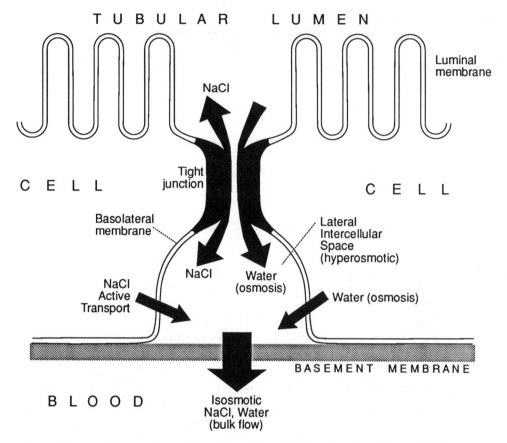

Figure 4–3. Paracellular pathway for sodium chloride and water movement in the proximal tubule.

space that forces fluid through the basement membrane and into the peritubular space, where Starling forces interact to move fluid and solutes across the peritubular capillaries (Fig. 4–3). This influence of peritubular capillary hydraulic and oncotic pressure on proximal tubular reabsorption represents an important mechanism for controlling sodium reabsorption.

Loop of Henle
The loop of Henle reabsorbs about 25% of the filtered sodium salts and 15% of the filtered water. This suggests that the loop is diluting the urine.

How can this occur if water is closely coupled to salt transport? The answer was provided by microperfusion studies demonstrating major differences in the permeability of descending and ascending thin limbs. In contrast to most tissues, there is poor correlation between solute and water permeability in the loop of Henle. Instead, **water permeability is very high in the thin descending limb and very low in the thin ascending limb** (Fig. 4–4). **Solute permeabilities are low in**

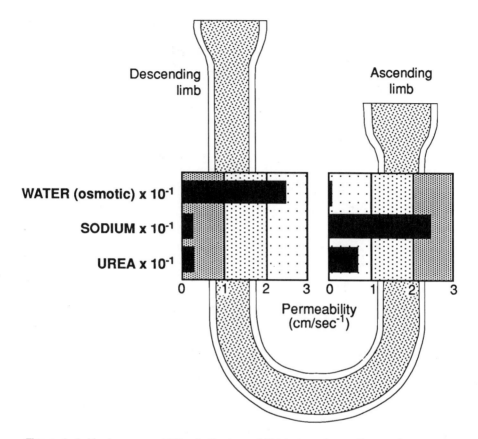

Figure 4–4. Varying permeabilities in the loop of Henle to water, sodium, and urea. *(From Kokko JP, Tisher CC: Water movement across nephron segments involved with the count or current muliplication system. Kidney Int. 1976; 10:64–68.)*

the descending limb but very high for sodium chloride and moderately high for urea in the ascending limb.

In contrast to most nephron segments, the transtubular electrical potential is **positive in the lumen** during microperfusion studies as long as sodium chloride is present in the perfusate and bath. The lumen-positive PD is the result of the net excess of anions crossing the cell and passive diffusion of potassium into the lumen. A schema of tubular transport in this segment based on in vitro studies is shown in Figure 4–5.

A major consequence of the large lumen-positive gradient in the thick ascending limb is the passive transcellular movement of calcium and magnesium ions into the interstitium. Loop diuretics (furosemide, bumetanide, ethacrynic acid) block active luminal transport and produce a loss of calcium and magnesium as well as sodium chloride. Clinically, this observation is used to treat diseases in which excesses of calcium and magnesium are present.

L u m e n   C e l l   I n t e r s t i t u m

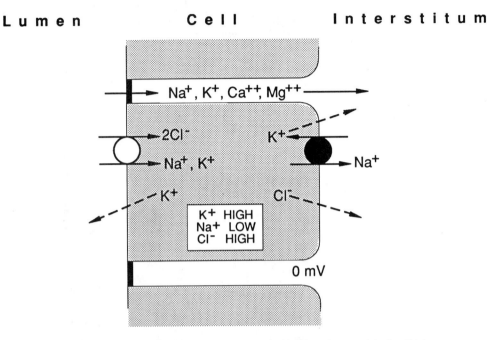

Figure 4–5. Schema of sodium, potassium, and chloride cotransport in the thick ascending limb of the loop of Henle. Solid lines represent active transport, and dotted lines represent passive transport.

Distal Convoluted Tubule

The distal convoluted tubule (DCT) is relatively impermeable to urea and water. Active sodium transport is the primary process, and the lumen-negative voltage generated provides a driving force for chloride transport, which is mostly passive. The junctional tightness of this segment prevents much paracellular backflux of solutes despite the large gradients created. Thus, tubular fluid continues to be diluted by solute removal without regard to the water requirements of the body.

The macula densa separates the thick ascending limb from the true DCT. This specialized tubular segment, the afferent and efferent arterioles, and the extraglomerular mesangium form the juxtaglomerular apparatus (see Chapter 1). **Macula densa cells somehow act as sensors of sodium salt balance** and send a signal to the granular cells in the afferent arterioles. When the sodium chloride concentration in the distal tubule is low, renin release occurs, angiotensin increases, and aldosterone is stimulated with subsequent sodium conservation.

The DCT and collecting segments respond to the action of aldosterone. Hypoaldosteronism leads to a decreased rate of tubular sodium chloride reabsorption and depletion of total body sodium. This imbalance is correctable by the administration of aldosterone analogs, such as fludrocortisone.

The Collecting Tubules

Fluid entering the cortical collecting tubule is dilute, coming as it does from the thick ascending limb and DCT, where solute is reabsorbed without water.

This segment of the nephron is the final site of regulation of urinary sodium, potassium, hydrogen ions (protons or acid), and water excretion. Transport in these tubular segments is similar to that in the DCT, but it differs in showing physiologic responses to several hormones. Although the quantity of sodium transported is small, a high tubular fluid/plasma concentration ratio (TF/P) can be achieved. During conditions requiring sodium and water retention, urinary osmolarity can rise to three or four times that of plasma, and urinary sodium concentration can be reduced to almost zero.

SODIUM BALANCE: REGULATION OF THE EXTRACELLULAR VOLUME

Sodium Balance

Sodium Determines Extracellular Fluid (ECF) Volume. The principal solute in the ECF is sodium and its attendant anions. The concentration of these salts in the ECF determines the effective osmotic pressure of the interstitial fluid and, hence, cellular hydration. There are about 80 mmol/kg in a normal adult, or about 5600 mmol of sodium in a 70 kg individual. About 40% of this body sodium is in the ECF. A large amount of sodium is contained in bone, but only half of this is freely exchangeable with sodium in the ECF (Fig. 4–6).

Effects of Increased Sodium Intake. The average person ingests about 150 mmol (range 100 to 300 mmol) of sodium salts daily. With a constant intake of sodium, a comparable amount is excreted each day, mostly in the urine, with a variable amount in sweat and a small fraction in the feces.

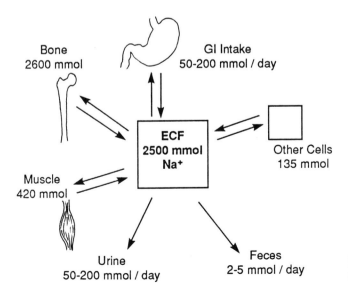

Figure 4–6. Sodium balance in an adult.

If sodium intake exceeds excretion, body salt balance increases (often called positive balance). This might be a short-term imbalance resulting from a salty meal or a chronic imbalance caused by renal, heart, or liver dysfunction.

Renal Responses to Changes in Dietary Sodium Intake. It is obvious from reviewing Figure 4–6 that the major regulators of sodium balance are dietary intake and renal excretion. The usual renal responses to a change in sodium intake are depicted in Figure 4–7.

If a normal subject on a constant daily intake of 100 mmol/day of sodium reduces the sodium intake to about 10 mmol/day, a progressive decrease of urine sodium excretion occurs. After 4 or 5 days, sodium excretion is again approximately equivalent to dietary intake. During the period of negative sodium balance, weight falls by approximately 1.5 to 2 kg (due to a reduction of the ECF volume) and then levels off as a new steady state occurs. **During these adjustments, the normal subject is asymptomatic, and there is no change in serum chemistries.**

If this same subject then increases the sodium intake to 200 mmol/day, the reverse of the previous events occurs. That is, over the next 3 to 5 days, urinary

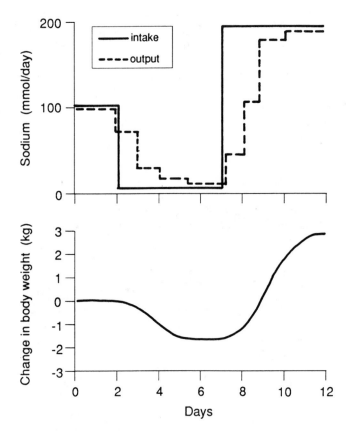

Figure 4–7. Normal response to variations in sodium intake.

sodium excretion slowly rises to equal sodium intake. Concomitant with this positive sodium balance, body weight rises and exceeds the original level because of a slightly expanded ECF volume. Thus, **the kidney is capable of varying sodium output over a wide range in response to dietary alterations, with only modest changes in ECF volume.**

Renal Control Mechanisms. Since there is no physiologic regulation of sodium intake in humans, balance must be achieved by regulating renal sodium excretion to match intake. How does the kidney perceive changes in sodium balance and adjust its excretion appropriately? Sodium is freely filterable at the glomerulus and actively reabsorbed but not secreted by the tubules. Thus, the amount of sodium excreted in the urine represents a balance between two processes, glomerular filtration and tubular reabsorption.

$$\text{Sodium excretion} = \text{sodium filtered } - \text{ sodium reabsorbed}$$
$$= (\text{GRF} \times [\text{Na}]_p) \ - \text{ sodium reabsorbed}$$

In theory, it is possible to adjust sodium excretion by controlling any of these three variables. In reality, however, the plasma sodium concentration is maintained within relatively narrow limits. Therefore, sodium excretion mainly depends on the reflex control of GFR and sodium reabsorption. Sodium excretion could be raised greatly by elevating the GFR and simultaneously reducing reabsorption. Conversely, sodium excretion could be decreased below normal levels by lowering the GFR and raising sodium reabsorption.

Regulation of renal sodium excretion involves input sensors that detect the ECF volume and output responses that produce changes in salt handling by the kidney. On the input side, alterations in plasma volume are monitored both on the venous side (stretch receptors in the great veins and atria) and arterial effective volume that is filling the arterial circulation by the cardiac output. Central nervous system response to baroreceptor signals and the release of several hormonal factors influence tubular sodium regulation. **In addition to neurogenic and hormonal influences, the arterial blood pressure and the physical properties of blood (hematocrit, plasma protein concentration) directly affect the excretion of salt by the kidney.**

Control of Glomerular Filtration Rate (GFR)

With a stable plasma sodium concentration, changes in GFR could markedly alter the filtered load of sodium and lead to striking changes in sodium excretion if tubular reabsorption remained constant. This is not the case, however, for two reasons.

First, under normal conditions, **GFR is kept relatively constant by autoregulation.**

Second, **in the absence of changes in ECF volume, modulations in tubular reabsorption match changes in GFR.** This phenomenon, known as **glomerulotubular balance,** prevents even large changes in GFR from altering sodium excretion. This coupling between mechanisms for renal sodium control must affect tubular reabsorption independently from the GFR. This relationship is seen clearly in patients with chronic renal disease and a falling GFR. Despite diminution in filtered sodium, patients usually maintain normal sodium excretion by decreasing tubular sodium reabsorption (Fig. 4–8).

Control of Sodium Reabsorption

Experience has shown that **expansion of ECF volume depresses renal sodium reabsorption. Conversely, ECF volume contraction enhances renal sodium reabsorption.** Hormonal, peritubular Starling forces and neurogenic factors are all involved in these processes.

Hormonal Regulation of Sodium Excretion. Multiple hormones are involved in regulation of renal sodium excretion, including aldosterone, angiotensin II, prostaglandins, bradykinin, and natriuretic hormones.

Aldosterone. This hormone is the best studied effector of renal sodium balance. **Sodium reabsorption is stimulated primarily in the cortical collecting tubules.** Angiotensin is the dominant stimulus for aldosterone biosynthesis in the adrenal gland, but ACTH and other stimuli for aldosterone secretion include an increase in

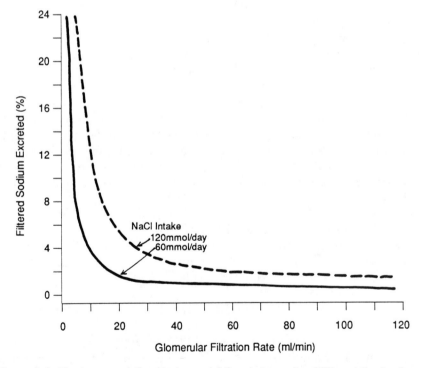

Figure 4–8. The inverse relationship in renal failure between the GFR and the fraction of filtered sodium excreted in the urine.

serum potassium, a fall in blood volume or serum sodium, and a rise in estrogen concentration. Tubular action results from at least three factors: increases in the enzymes available for ATP synthesis; increased sodium permeability of the luminal membrane, and increases in Na–K-ATPase in the basolateral membrane. Although the total quantity of sodium reabsorption dependent on the influence of aldosterone is probably less than 5% of the filtered load, this amount is highly significant in view of the large amount of sodium filtered daily. Actually, excretion of 1% of the filtered load of sodium in a normal subject represents more than the average sodium intake and would cause sodium depletion. In addition to its effect on sodium transport, aldosterone increases urinary excretion of potassium and hydrogen ions.

Angiotensin II. **Renin released from afferent arterioles increases conversion of angiotensinogen to angiotensin I, which in turn is rapidly converted to angiotensin II.** Effects on renal sodium transport include **stimulation of adrenal release of aldosterone, intrarenal vasoconstriction, and direct stimulation of proximal tubule reabsorption. From the viewpoint of total body sodium economy, aldosterone stimulation is the most significant action.**

Prostaglandins. **These extremely active vasodilators are produced within the kidney** and modulate renal hemodynamics and salt and water balance. They **decrease sodium chloride absorption** and oppose various intrarenal vasoconstrictive mechanisms.

Natriuretic Hormones. Acute volume expansion or an increase in sodium intake produces both increased sodium excretion by inhibiting sodium reabsorption and increased vascular tone. More than one circulating substance is responsible for these changes. One recently identified hormone, atrial natriuretic factor (ANF), is short-acting and produces its diuretic action by relaxing renal arterioles and increasing GFR, inhibiting sodium transport in the collecting ducts, and reducing the circulating concentration of renin, aldosterone, and ADH.

Peritubular Starling Forces. Hydraulic and protein oncotic pressures are fundamental in regulating movement of fluid and solute across all systemic capillaries. The kidney, however, is unique in two ways.

Peritubular capillary oncotic pressure is higher than systemic capillary oncotic pressure (35 to 45 versus 20 to 30 mm Hg). This occurs because 20% to 30% of the plasma fluid is removed in the glomerulus by filtration before reaching the peritubular capillaries. The increase in oncotic pressure depends on the fraction of the renal plasma flow that is filtered by the glomerulus. This filtration fraction varies continuously depending on the degree of renal arteriolar constriction.

The **hydraulic pressure in the peritubular capillaries** is considerably lower than in most systemic capillaries (10 to 15 versus 20 to 25 mm Hg) because of the vascular resistance caused by both afferent and efferent arterioles.

Both factors tend to enhance the reabsorption of salt and water by the

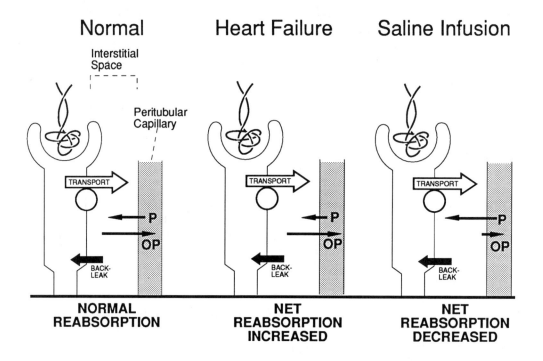

Figure 4–9. Influence of peritubular capillary hydraulic pressure (P) and plasma oncotic pressure (OP) on net tubular reabsorption.

proximal and distal tubules. When renal sodium retention occurs because of ECF volume depletion or a disease that produces edema, there is an increase in both the renal resistance and the filtration fraction. Thus, hydraulic pressure will be reduced and oncotic pressure will be increased in peritubular capillaries, enhancing reabsorption of fluid.

Conversely, renal vasodilation (as might occur after increased ingestion of salt and water) would be associated with a decreased filtration fraction, a higher hydraulic pressure, a smaller than normal rise in peritubular capillary oncotic pressure, and, therefore, less sodium reabsorption (Fig. 4–9).

Adrenergic Nervous System. The direct influences of adrenergic factors on sodium transport have been difficult to separate from hemodynamic effects. Renal denervation produces a prompt increase in sodium excretion, whereas intrarenal infusions of catecholamines cause vasoconstriction and a decrease in sodium excretion. Conversely, low doses of dopamine, an epinephrine precursor, increase sodium excretion. It is likely that the final renal action of these substances is a combination of hemodynamic and direct tubular effects.

SAMPLE ANSWERS TO STUDY QUESTIONS

1. Write the equation relating filtration, reabsorption, and excretion of sodium.

Excretion = filtration − reabsorbtion
T_S = (GFR × $[Na]_S$) − ($[Na]_u$ × V), where
T_S = tubular transport of substance **S**
GFR = glomerular filtration rate
$[Na]_s$ = serum sodium concentration
$[Na]_u$ = urinary sodium concentration
V = urine flow rate

2. For each 150 mmol of sodium chloride or sodium bicarbonate reabsorbed by the proximal tubule, how much water is reabsorbed?

The salt and water reabsorption in the proximal tubule is in isosmotic proportions (150 mmol NaCl or $NaHCO_3$/L of solution). Hence, approximately 1 L of water will be transported with each 150 mmol of NaCl or $NaHCO_3$ that is reabsorbed.

3. Where is the site of osmotic equilibration between solutes and water in the proximal tubule?

According to current concepts, equilibration occurs in the intercellular space. The sodium chloride mainly comes from the intracellular space, and water movement occurs by osmotic flow across the cell and tight junction.

4. How does mannitol, an osmotic diuretic, inhibit the recovery of salt and water in the proximal tubule?

Because proximal tubular fluid always remains isosmotic to cortical plasma, mannitol, a nonreabsorbed solute, sequesters water by osmotic flow in the tubular lumen. Since the proximal tubule can only pump sodium against a small gradient (maximal gradient about 100 mmol/L), not all of the sodium is pumped out of the water that is retained by mannitol. Consequently, the reabsorption of both salt and water is reduced in comparison to normal conditions in this segment. The net result is diuresis, with increased excretion of salt and water in the urine.

5. Compare salt and water transport in the proximal tubule with that in the thick ascending limb and the collecting duct.

In the proximal tubule, water transport is closely coupled to active sodium transport, whereas in the thick ascending limb, very little water gets reabsorbed. In the collecting duct, sodium and water transport occur but are independent of each other.

6. **Calculate the fractional sodium excretion (percent of the filtered sodium excreted) from the following data:**
   $[sodium]_p$ = 144 mmol/L
   $[sodium]_u$ = 200 mmol/L
   urine flow = 36 mL/30min
   Cl_{inulin} = 120 mL/min = 0.12 L/min

   Filtered sodium load = plasma sodium x inulin clearance
   Filtered Na load = 144 mmol/L $\times$ 0.12 L/min = 17.3 mmol/min

   Urine flow = 36 mL/30 min = 1.2 mL/min

   Urine sodium excretion = Urine sodium x urine flow rate
   Urine Na excreted = 200 mmol/L x 1.2 mL/min = 0.24 mmol/min

   Fractional sodium excretion = Urine Na/Filtered Na load
   Fractional Na excretion = 0.24/17.3 = 0.013 or 1.3%

7. **A normal adult reduces daily sodium ingestion from 150 to 10 mmol. Describe the sequential daily changes in:**
   a. body weight
   b. ECF volume
   c. serum sodium concentration
   d. daily urinary sodium excretion

   The reduction of daily sodium in the diet from 150 to 10 mmol/d would be followed by a reduction in body weight of several kilograms over a period of 3 to 5 days. The weight loss is due principally to a loss of isotonic extracellular fluid and, therefore, the ECF volume would decrease about 2 to 3 liters. Because a reduction in dietary sodium has no significant effect on osmolar regulation or thirst, no change would be seen in the serum sodium concentration. The daily urine sodium would decrease over the same period of time until a new steady state was achieved in which the dietary intake and urinary excretion of sodium were comparable.

8. **Describe the same changes noted in question 7 in a patient with renal failure (Cl_{cr} = 10 mL/min) whose dietary sodium is reduced from 150 to 10 mmol/day.**

   In contrast to the patient with normal renal function who can reduce his urinary sodium excretion to negligible amounts, the patient with renal insufficiency has an obligatory loss of sodium caused by osmotic diuresis in the residual functioning nephrons. In the patient with a creatinine clearance of 10 mL/min, the basal sodium excretion with no dietary intake will be about 30 to 50 mmol/d. Therefore, a diet with only 10 mmol/d will be less than the ongoing sodium loss and will lead to continuing weight loss and extracellular volume depletion. If continued, such a diet will lead to a marked contraction of the blood volume, a fall in cardiac output, and a further deterioration of renal function.

Concentration and Dilution

INTRODUCTION

The kidney maintains the equilibrium between intake and excretion of water by concentrating or diluting the urine. Because there are large variations in fluid intake as well as nonrenal losses (eg, sweating with exercise and high temperature, gastrointestinal losses), the kidney must be able to adjust its output widely. In fact, the normal kidney can vary the urine output from 500 ml to over 15,000 mL/day if necessary. This chapter deals with the mechanisms involved in the process of concentrating and diluting the urine.

STUDY QUESTIONS

1. Describe the properties of the nephron that cause the fluid entering the distal tubule to be dilute.
2. The desert kangaroo rat can concentrate urine to greater than 3000 mOsm/L, whereas maximum urine osmolarity in an amphibian is only 230 mOsm/L (isosmolarity for this species). What renal structural differences from humans would you postulate might be found in these two species to explain such a contrast in urinary concentrating ability?
3. Contrast the osmolarity and urine flow rate along the uriniferous tubule (proximal, loop, distal, collecting duct) in both the absence and the presence of vasopressin (antidiuretic hormone).
4. You are asked to evaluate a patient with a recent history of polyuria (increased urine flow). Daily urine volumes are 5 to 7 L, with an osmolarity of 125 to 200 mOsm/L. Describe what tests you would use to evaluate the cause of this abnormality and the physiologic meanings of any positive or negative findings.
5. Based on your personal experience and current understanding of human physiology, complete the graph in Figure 5–1, which correlates the temporal relationship between urine flow and osmolarity in a normal adult after oral ingestion of 1 L of water at time zero (note arrow on graph). Do not be concerned with absolute numbers but rather the general trend of increases and decreases over the 5 hour period.
6. Define
   a. Free water reabsorption
   b. Free water clearance

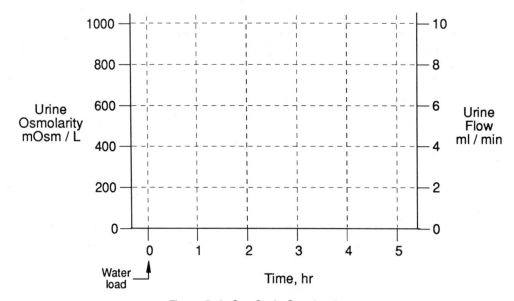

Figure 5–1. See Study Question 5.

TABLE 5–1. NORMAL WATER BALANCE IN ADULTS

Intake mL/day		Output mL/day	
Drunk	1200	Urine	1500
In food	1000	Sensible	50
Metabolically		Insensible	850
produced	300	Feces	100
Total	2500	Total	2500

GENERAL CONCEPTS

Intake and Output

On a daily basis, the intake and loss of water are equal. The two basic sources of water are **ingestion** (liquids and solid food) and **metabolism** (largely from carbohydrates). Water losses can occur through four routes: urine, gastrointestinal, skin, and lungs (Table 5–1).

Sensible Versus Insensible Losses

1. Insensible losses. **The loss of solute-poor water from the skin and solute-free water from the lungs is called an insensible loss because it largely occurs undetected.**
2. Sensible losses. **Noticeable** skin losses as **sweat** are called **sensible losses.** Although losses **via the gut** usually are small, they can be severe when vomiting and diarrhea are present.

The Renal Response

Water intake and losses may vary widely from the typical value depending on availability, social occasion, and environmental conditions. Faced with such highly variable intake and loss, the **kidneys adjust their rate of water excretion over a broad range** (Table 5–2) through an elegant series of transport mechanisms **to maintain a constant body fluid osmolarity**.

STRUCTURE AND FUNCTION

General Features

Eighty percent of the glomerular filtrate has been reabsorbed by the beginning of the distal convoluted tubule independent of body water balance. Therefore, **ad-**

TABLE 5–2. RANGE OF URINE VOLUMES AND OSMOLARITIES IN ADULTS

Condition	Vasopressin	Volume L/day	Urine Osmolarity mOsm/L
Water loaded	Absent	10–20	50–100
Water deficit	Maximal	0.3–0.6	900–1200

justments in water balance must result from variable recovery of the remaining 20% of the originally filtered water in the distal convoluted tubule and collecting ducts. This is accomplished by

1. The **countercurrent multiplier and exchanger system**, a unique structural arrangement of the vasa recta, Henle's loop, and the collecting ducts
2. **Varying permeabilities to water** in the loop of Henle and collecting tubular segments
3. **Active reabsorption** of sodium chloride from luminal fluid

Countercurrent Multiplier

A simple example of a countercurrent multiplier system is the increased heating at the apex of a loop of pipe shown schematically in Figure 5–2. The arrangement of countercurrent flow in the U-shape (tubule) allows an increase in fluid tempera-

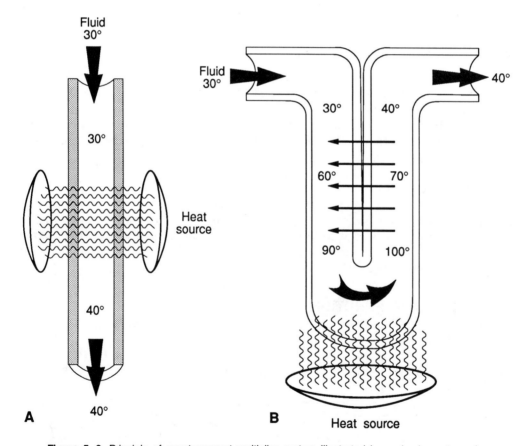

Figure 5–2. Principle of countercurrent multiplier system illustrated by a simple system of heating fluid. *(From Knox FG (ed):* Textbook of Renal Pathophysiology. *Hagerstown, Md: Harper & Row, 1978, p. 75.)*

ture (osmolarity) to a much higher level for any given increment of energy input than would be possible through single heating steps. There are three **basic requirements** for such a system to function as a renal countercurrent multiplier.

1. **Countercurrent flow,**
2. **Differences in permeability** between tubules carrying fluid in opposite directions, and
3. A source of **energy**.

As applied to the kidney (Fig. 5–3) (1) the loop of Henle provides countercurrent flow, (2) the descending limb is much more permeable to water than is the ascending limb, and (3) active transport of sodium chloride from the thick ascending limb to the surrounding interstitium provides the energy source.

The result of this arrangement is that the **luminal osmolarity is reduced within the ascending limb and simultaneously raised in the surrounding interstitial fluid.** Fluid that enters the descending limb initially is isosmotic with plasma but becomes more concentrated as water equilibrates across its permeable wall with the higher osmolarity of the interstitium. Fluid within the loops is then concentrated by the sequence of events illustrated in Figure 5–4.

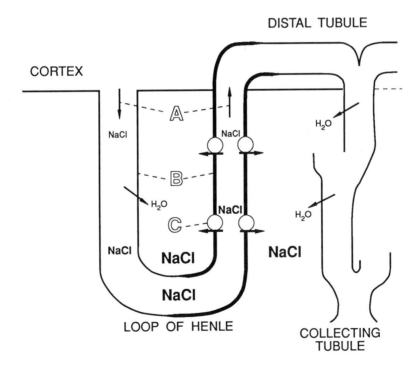

Figure 5–3. Countercurrent multiplication by the loop of Henle. Essential features are: **A,** countercurrent flow; **B,** differential permeabilities, **C,** energy source (ion pump). *(From Jamison RL, Maffly RH: The urinary concentrating mechanism. N Engl J Med. 1976; 295:1059.)*

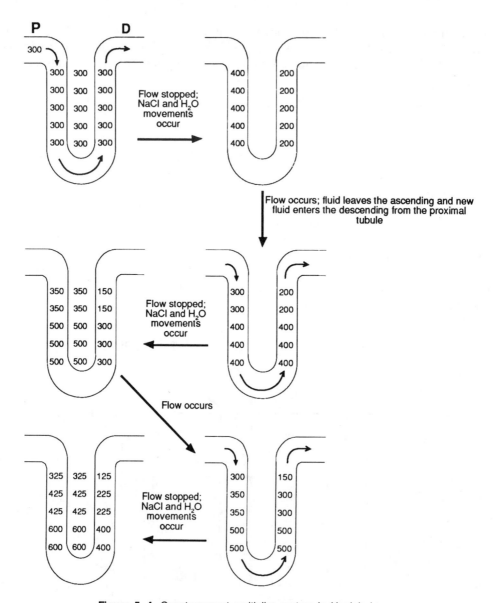

Figure 5–4. Countercurrent multiplier system in Henle's loop.

Thus, **the ability of the sodium chloride pump to establish a gradient across the wall of the ascending limb is multiplied by countercurrent flow to achieve a large osmotic difference**—approximately 900 mOsm/L in a dehydrated human—**between fluid in the proximal tubule and that in the tip of the papilla.**

Urea also makes a considerable contribution to the total osmolarity of the renal medulla. It diffuses along a concentration gradient into the interstitium from the late collecting duct and enters the ascending limb of the loop and possibly the descending limb of Henle's loop to complete the cycle. At a low dietary intake of protein, metabolic production of urea is reduced, leading to a decreased concentrating ability of the kidney.

Countercurrent Exchanger

Vasa Recta. The vasa recta are the medullary blood vessels. The looping U-shaped structures are similar in shape and run parallel to the loops of Henle. Straight vessels coursing through the medulla would reabsorb fluid and solutes and dissipate its elevated osmolarity. The vasa recta seem suitably **arranged to facilitate transcapillary exchange of nutrients, water, and solutes and still preserve the medullary osmotic gradient produced by the loops of Henle**. In this role, it is **called a countercurrent exchanger** (Fig. 5–5).

Transcapillary Forces in the Medulla. Outside of the renal medulla, solutes other than plasma proteins have little influence on fluid movement across capillaries. Only oncotic and hydraulic pressures are considered effective transcapillary driving forces. Nonprotein solutes exert minimal osmotic pressure because the concentrations in the interstitial fluid and plasma are very similar. However, conditions in

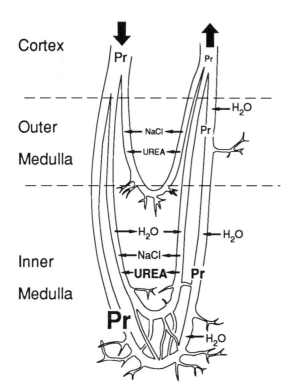

Figure 5–5. Countercurrent exchange by the vasa recta. **Pr** denotes plasma protein. The size of type indicates the relative concentrate of each solute with respect to its location in the medulla but not necessarily with respect to other solutes. The progressive rise in this concentration of sodium chloride and urea in the medullary interstitium is due to the loop of Henle and collecting tubule. Since the capillaries are permeable to sodium chloride and urea, these solutes enter descending vasa recta and leave ascending vasa recta. This transcapillary exchange helps trap the solutes in the medulla. *(From Jamison RL, Maffly RH: The urinary concentrating mechanism. N Engl J Med. 1976; 295:1059.)*

the medullary microcirculation are more complex. As blood enters the medulla in the **descending vasa recta**, the net transcapillary pressure favors fluid loss. In addition, there is a lag in osmotic equilibration across the vasa recta because of the relatively high blood flow rate (about two to three times greater than urine flow in the loop of Henle), so that the concentration of small solutes is slightly higher in the interstitium than in the plasma at the same level. This produces a transcapillary osmotic pressure that counters the plasma oncotic pressure and thus **exaggerates fluid loss in the descending vasa recta**. In contrast, as blood flows up the **ascending vasa recta**, the concentration of small solutes exceeds that in the adjacent interstitium, owing to a similar lag in osmotic equilibration—but now in the opposite direction—so that, instead of opposing each other, transcapillary osmotic and oncotic forces in the ascending vasa recta act in the same direction to **favor capillary fluid uptake**. In fact, fluid entry into the ascending vasa recta exceeds the volume of fluid lost from the descending vasa recta. The excess fluid entering capillaries represents net fluid removal from the medulla and is equal to the volume of fluid reabsorbed from the collecting ducts and descending limb of Henle. Thus the **osmolarity of the medulla is maintained by the vasa recta**.

ANTIDIURETIC HORMONE OR VASOPRESSIN

The osmolarity of ECF (280 to 300 mOsm/L) is maintained primarily by regulation of intake (thirst) and excretion of water by the kidneys. **Renal excretion is mainly under the control of vasopressin secretion**.

The neurohypophysis releases vasopressin in response to two factors, ECF osmolarity and ECF volume. It is most sensitive to ECF osmolarity, responding to changes of as little as 1%. In contrast, changes in ECF volume must be quite gross (probably greater than 5%) to stimulate vasopressin release. However, a volume stimulus overrides an osmolarity stimulus, often producing serious water imbalance.

Extracellular Fluid (ECF) Osmolarity
The relationship between changes in plasma osmolarity and vasopressin concentration in healthy adults is seen in Figure 5–6. Recent data indicate that the important stimulus for vasopressin release is the concentration of sodium in the cerebrospinal fluid (CSF) or extracellular space of the brain.

Extracellular Fluid Volume
How do changes in ECF volume mediate vasopressin release? Apparently, hypothalamic cells receive neurogenic stimuli from several **vascular baroreceptors**, particularly a group located in the left atrium. These stretch receptors are stimulated by changes in left atrial pressure. A decrease in ECF volume decreases left atrial pressure, stimulating vasopressin release.

Increased atrial pressure will have the opposite effect. It should be noted that

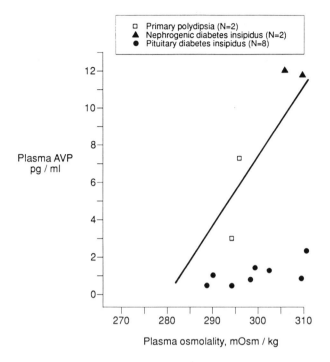

Figure 5–6. The relationship of plasma arginine vasopressin to plasma osmolarity in healthy adults and patients with different types of polyuria. The line represents multiple measurements from 25 normal adults. *(From Robertson GL, Shelton RL, Athar S: The osmoregulation of vasopressin.* Kidney Int. *1976; 10:25.)*

volume regulation of vasopressin release is an emergency system that operates only when severe derangements occur, such as volume depletion. In such circumstances, control of osmolarity is sacrificed to maintain adequate intravascular volume, but hyposmolarity occurs.

Miscellaneous Factors

In addition to osmolar and volume stimuli, vasopressin release may be influenced by other neurogenic stimuli (**fear, pain, anxiety**) as well as **drugs**. Most drugs that influence vasopressin are stimulatory, a few suppress secretion, and some change the renal response to vasopressin (Table 5–3).

WATER AND OSMOLAR CLEARANCE

Urine/Plasma (U/P) Osmolar Ratio

A qualitative assessment of whether the kidney is conserving or excreting water in excess of isosmolar solute excretion can be made by comparing the urine osmolarity with that of plasma. **A U/P osmolar ratio of greater than 1 indicates a concentrated urine and retention of water. A U/P osmolar ratio less than 1 indicates a dilute urine and excretion of excess water.**

TABLE 5–3. EXAMPLES OF AGENTS THAT INTERFERE WITH REGULATION OF RENAL HANDLING OF WATER

Mechanism	Decreasing renal diluting ability	Mechanism	Decreasing renal concentrating ability
Stimulation of vasopressin release	Nicotine Chlorpropamide Clofibrate Morphine Vincristine Carbamazepine	Suppressing vasopressin release	Ethanol Phenytoin Lithium
Sensitizing kidney to vasopressin or mimicking vasopressin effect	Chlorpropamide Biguanides Acetaminophen Oxytocin Chlorothiazide	Reducing kidney responsiveness to vasopressin	Demeclocycline Lithium

Free Water Clearance

A more quantitative evaluation of excretion and conservation of water can be made by measurement of free water clearance (C_{H_2O}). It is unfortunate that such terminology has become embedded in medical literature because free water clearance is not really a true clearance at all but **denotes the volume of pure water (water free of solute) that would need to be removed from the urine to make it isosmolar to plasma**. The equation for calculating free water clearance is:

$$C_{H_2O} = V - Cl_{osm}$$

Where V is the urine volume per unit time and Cl_{osm} is the osmolar clearance. The osmolar clearance is calculated in a conventional manner

$$Cl_{osm} = \frac{(osm)_u \times V}{(osm)_p}$$

These equations indicate that

1. C_{H_2O} is zero when the U/P osmolar ratio is 1
2. When urine has a greater osmolarity than plasma, C_{H_2O} is negative (or Tc_{H_2O}, free water reabsorption, is positive)
3. **Maximum C_{H_2O} measured during a water diuresis is about 10 to 15 mL/min; this represents an ability to excrete 15 to 20 L daily of free water.**
4. **During water conservation, the maximum negative C_{H_2O} is 1 to 2 mL/min; this represents the ability to conserve 2 to 3 L of free water daily**

THE END RESULT: DILUTION AND CONCENTRATION

Dilution of Urine

Ascending Limb of Henle's Loop = ***"The Diluting Segment."*** Micropuncture studies show that the **fluid entering the distal convoluted tubule is always hyposmolar** to plasma regardless of the state of water balance (Fig. 5–7). Since the proximal tubule reabsorbs salt and water isosmotically and fluid in the early distal tubule is always hyposmolar to plasma, dilution must occur in the loop of Henle. Recent studies of isolated, perfused tubules indicate that the thick ascending limb of Henle's loop is responsible for producing dilute tubular fluid. **It possesses a large capacity for active sodium chloride reabsorption and a very low water permeability that is not altered by vasopressin.** No other segment of the nephron shares this combination of properties, and this segment is often called the **diluting segment.** It should be noted that all nephrons produce a dilute urine in the early distal tubule regardless of whether or not they possess short or long loops of

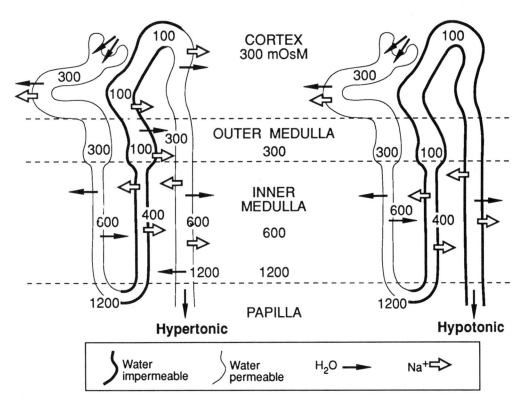

Figure 5–7. Changes in tubular fluid osmolarity in the presence (left) and absence (right) of vasopressin.

Henle. In contrast, only the juxtamedullary nephrons with long loops participate in the urinary concentration mechanism.

Absence of Vasopressin Leads to Dilute Urine. Vasopressin controls the **water permeability of the cortical collecting tubules and medullary collecting ducts**. When vasopressin is absent or reduced, as in diabetes insipidus, these segments are impermeable to water, and urine osmolarity is low (50 to 100 mOsm/L), differing very little from the fluid leaving the diluting segment. Urine flow rates of 15 to 20 L daily (about 10% of the glomerular filtrate) may occur. These observations indicate that **very little water reabsorption occurs in the distal nephron and collecting segments when vasopressin is absent**. Similar urine flow rates and osmolarity are observed in individuals who have ingested rapidly as little as 1 L of water, which represents a dilution of body fluids of about 2%. Evidently, small decreases in body fluid osmolarity are sufficient to inhibit vasopressin release.

Concentration of Urine

Establishment of Hypertonic Interstitium. Conservation of body water is largely the task of the kidneys, allowing survival when water is not readily available. Concentration of urine by the kidneys involves the complex structural and functional interactions that permit water reabsorption to be coupled to active solute transport described previously. The analogy of the arrangement of Henle's loop to a countercurrent heat exchanger pointed out how small differences in solute concentration between fluid flowing in the ascending and descending limbs of the loop of Henle could result in very large differences in solute concentration along the length of the tubules and the surrounding interstitium.

Water Reabsorption: Concentrating the Urine. **In the presence of large amounts of vasopressin, the collecting tubules and collecting ducts are completely permeable to water.** Thus, **water moves freely into the surrounding interstitium** and the osmolarity in the collecting duct can be as high as that in the medullary interstitium (1200 mOsm/L). With lower vasopressin levels, the tubules are less permeable, less water is reabsorbed, and the urine osmolarity will be somewhat below the maximum, as the body's requirements dictate.

SAMPLE ANSWERS TO STUDY QUESTIONS

1. **Describe the properties of the nephron that cause the fluid entering the distal tubule to be dilute.**

   The thick ascending limb actively absorbs sodium chloride but has a very low water permeability that is not altered by vasopressin. As a result, the fluid entering the distal convoluted tubule is dilute (approximately 100 mOsm/L).

2. **The desert kangaroo rat can concentrate urine to greater than 3000 mOsm/ L, whereas maximum urine osmolarity in an amphibian is only 230 mOsm/L (isosmolarity for this species). What renal structural differences from humans would you postulate might be found in these two species to explain such a contrast in urinary concentrating ability?**

   Because the capacity to concentrate urine is intimately related to the medullary countercurrent system, one would suspect that the desert kangaroo rat can concentrate well because of an increased number of juxtamedullary nephrons with long medullary loops. In fact, almost all of the cortical nephrons in this animal are juxtamedullary in type, and the loops of Henle are long. The medullary cross-sectional width is fivefold greater than the cortical width.

   On the other hand, the amphibian has a very small medulla, with no thin loops of Henle. This animal lives in a moist environment and has little need to conserve water. Urine flow rate is controlled mainly by changes in GFR. Both amphibian skin and bladder respond to vasopressin, which aids in maintaining water balance in this species.

3. **Contrast the osmolarity and urine flow rate along the uriniferous tubule (proximal, loop, distal, collecting duct) in both the absence and the presence of vasopressin (antidiuretic hormone).**

   The only areas of the uriniferous tubule that are sigificantly affected by vasopressin are the cortical and medullary collecting tubule and duct. Active solute transport continues in the distal uriniferous tubule and, in the absence of vasopressin, results in a dilute urine of 50 to 75 mOsm/L. When vasopressin is present in high titers and solute excretion is modest, the urine may approach the osmolarity of the papilla, about 1200 mOsm/L.

4. **You are asked to evaluate a patient with a recent history of polyuria (increased urine flow). Daily urine volumes are 5 to 7 L, with an osmolarity of 125 to 200 mOsm/L. Describe what tests you would use to evaluate the cause of this abnormality and the physiologic meanings of any positive or negative findings.**

   Polyuria in an adult is defined as a daily urine volume exceeding 2.5 L. Polyuria could be related to compulsive water drinking, with suppression of vasopressin release, pituitary disease with lack of vasopressin synthesis or release, or nephrogenic factors that prevent a normal response to vasopressin.

   Patients with compulsive water drinking usually have mild to moderate reduction in serum osmolarity as a result of a large water intake. In addition, they respond with urinary concentration when water is withheld for 4 to 6 hours.

   If a patient continues to have polyuria despite water restriction, weight loss will occur and plasma osmolarity will rise. At this point, parenteral vasopressin can be given. If the polyuria stops, pituitary disease with vasopressin deficiency is present (central diabetes insipidus). If polyuria persists despite the administration of vasopressin, the cause must be renal resistance to vasopressin (so-called nephrogenic diabetes insipidus).

5. **Based on your personal experience and current understanding of human physiology, complete the graph in Figure 5–1, which correlates the temporal relationship between urine flow and osmolarity in a normal adult after oral ingestion of 1 L of water at time zero (note arrow on graph). Do not be concerned with absolute numbers but rather the general trend of increases and decreases over the 5 hour period.**

Following oral ingestion of a water load of this quantity, a measurable small decrease in plasma osmolarity would occur in about 30 to 60 minutes (Fig. 5–8). Vasopressin release would be inhibited, and the normal residual circulating vasopressin would be eliminated slowly over a period of approximately 1 hour. This would result in a peak urine flow rate at about 90 minutes after the water load. The flow rate probably would be in the vicinity of 5 to 10 mL/min at this time, with a urine osmolarity in the vicinity of 100 mOsm/L. There would then be a gradual fall in urine flow rate and a rise in urine osmolarity over the next 3 to 6 hours.

6. **Define**
   a. Free water reabsorption
   b. Free water clearance

Free water reabsorption is water reabsorbed by the kidney when the urine is concentrated. For instance, if in 24 hours a patient excretes 500 mL of urine concentrated to 1200 mOsm/L (600 mOsm in 500 mL), approximately 1.5 L of

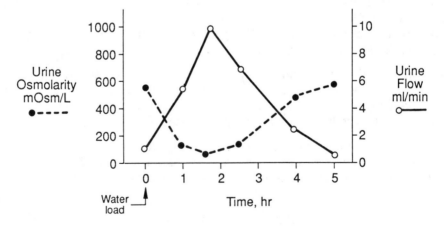

Figure 5–8. Answer 5 illustrated.

solute-free water has been reabsorbed. This results from the fact that if the urine were at the same osmolarity (about 300 mOsm/L) as plasma (no free water reabsorption), it would require 2000 mL to eliminate the solute load.

Free water clearance represents the excess water excreted when the urine is dilute. If a patient excretes 6000 mL containing 600 mOsm (100 mOsm/L), he has eliminated 4000 mL of free water in excess of the amount needed to maintain body osmolarity constant.

Renal Handling of Potassium

INTRODUCTION

This chapter discusses the renal mechanisms that control potassium balance in health. Potassium is the principal cation of the intracellular fluid. Severe imbalance may cause life-threatening cardiac or neuromuscular dysfunction. Potassium balance is affected by both external factors, such as diet, and internal factors, such as acid-base balance, adrenergic stimuli, and urine flow rate.

STUDY QUESTIONS

1. Based on the concepts presented in this chapter, what fraction of filtered potassium is present at each of the following tubular sites?

Site	Diet		
	Normal(%)	K deficiency (%)	K excess (%)
Beginning of proximal tubule	_____	_____	_____
End of proximal tubule	_____	_____	_____
Early distal tubule	_____	_____	_____
Ureteral urine	_____	_____	_____
(fractional excretion)	_____	_____	_____

The following data pertain to Questions 2,3, and 4. A woman with end-stage renal disease (ESRD) had the following laboratory results.

- 24 hour urine volume = 2.8 L
- [Creatinine]$_u$ = 32 mg/dL
- [Creatinine]$_p$ = 12.5 mg/dL
- [Potassium]$_u$ = 28.6 mmol/L
- [Potassium]$_p$ = 6.0 mmol/L

2. Calculate the fractional excretion of potassium (C_{K^+}/GFR).
3. What do these results indicate about potassium renal transport that is not demonstrable in a healthy subject?
4. Based on current physiologic concepts, what factors could have produced the potassium fractional excretion data noted in the patient?
5. You are consulted about a patient with persistent hypokalemia (serum K<3 mmol/L). What **single** test would you obtain to confirm renal versus nonrenal causes for this problem?
6. Hypokalemia and total body potassium depletion are part of the clinical picture of primary aldosteronism. What two dietary changes would help correct this abnormality? Explain the rationale for your answer.

INTRARENAL POTASSIUM TRANSPORT

Compared to oral potassium intake (50 to 100 mmol daily), the quantity of potassium filtered by the kidney is very large. **Between 700 and 800 mmol of potassium typically pass through the glomeruli daily in healthy adults.**

$$\text{GFR} = 180\text{L/day}$$
$$\text{Plasma potassium} = [K^+]_p = 4 \text{ mmol/L}$$
$$\text{Filtered } K^+ = \text{GFR} \times [K^+]_p$$
$$\text{Filtered } K^+ = 180 \text{ L/day} \times 4 \text{ mmol/L}$$
$$\text{Filtered } K^+ = 720 \text{ mmol/day}$$

Because the amount of potassium excreted in the urine is usually a small fraction (10 to 15%) of the filtered amount, **net tubular reabsorption must occur.** When certain conditions are present (high potassium diet, severe renal failure), net secretion also can be demonstrated because the excreted quantity of potassium exceeds that which is filtered. Thus, potassium transport is bidirectional, both **reabsorption and secretion are present simultaneously.**

Micropuncture evidence suggests that potassium is filtered freely by the glomerulus, undergoes net reabsorption in the proximal tubule and loop of Henle, and is reabsorbed or secreted in the distal collecting tubule and duct. The degree and direction of distal transport depends on multiple factors, such as the amount of fluid and salts reaching the distal tubule, acid-base status, potassium balance, and aldosterone concentration.

Proximal Tubule

Transport can be either passive or active. The major force for potassium in this segment is the **transepithelial potential difference** (PD). In the late proximal tubule, a lumen-positive gradient favors reabsorption. Micropuncture data demonstrate that 40% to 60% of filtered potassium is reabsorbed (Fig. 6–1) independent of changes in diet.

Loop of Henle

Potassium shows net reabsorption in this segment. Although measurements from deep loops at their turning point show a fractional amount of potassium that exceeds the filtered load by 13% as a consequence of secretion into the descending limb, net reabsorption occurs because of considerable absorption in the thick ascending limb as a result of a Na^+, K^+, $2Cl^-$ symporter (Fig. 4–5, a carrier mechanism that transports two or more different ions simultaneously through a membrane).

Distal Collecting Tubule and Duct

In contrast to prior nephron segments, **potassium transport in the distal nephron cannot be attributed to passive mechanisms**, although the lumen-negative PD in the late collecting tubules favors secretion. Studies have clearly shown **potassium reabsorption and secretion to occur in these segments.** A low potassium diet leads to net reabsorption, whereas a high potassium diet brings about net secretion.

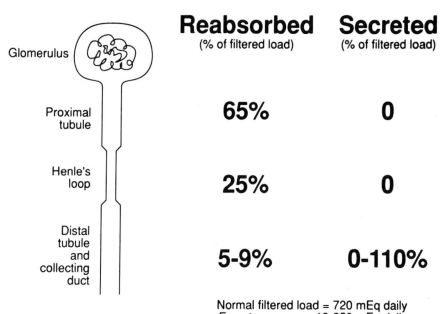

	Reabsorbed (% of filtered load)	Secreted (% of filtered load)
Glomerulus		
Proximal tubule	65%	0
Henle's loop	25%	0
Distal tubule and collecting duct	5-9%	0-110%

Normal filtered load = 720 mEq daily
Excretory range = 10-850 mEq daily

Figure 6–1. Potassium handling along the nephron.

Thus, dietary influences on potassium balance are modulated by transport changes in the distal nephron. Reabsorption is thought to operate at a basal level, and variations that control potassium balance are governed by secretion.

CONTROL OF POTASSIUM SECRETION

Most potassium excretion results from secretion in the distal collecting tubules and ducts. Microperfusion studies demonstrate that potassium depletion induces a decreased potassium flux across luminal and peritubular membranes and a fall in exchangeable intracellular potassium. Opposite changes follow potassium loading, infusion of bicarbonate, sodium deprivation, and administration of aldosterone.

In summary, there are **four major influences** on renal potassium secretion: (1) **plasma potassium concentration,** (2) **aldosterone levels,** (3) **acid-base balance,** and (4) **the delivery of fluid and poorly absorbable anions to the distal tubule.**

Plasma Potassium Concentration
Distal tubular potassium secretion is directly proportional to potassium intake and plasma concentration. This probably reflects changes in intracellular potassium concentration. For example, increased ingestion of potassium increases distal tubular secretion. The following sequence of events may occur: (1) an increase in extracellular concentration with an enhanced peritubular uptake, (2) an increase in aldosterone secretion secondary to an increased plasma potassium concentration— the elevated aldosterone titers also enhance peritubular potassium uptake, and (3) the resultant increase in intracellular potassium in distal tubular cells enhances the gradient for secretion into the lumen. The opposite sequence of events occurs with a negative potassium balance because of inadequate dietary intake or excessive gastrointestinal or renal losses:(1) a lowered extracellular concentration leads to (2) a low intracellular concentration and (3) a reduced aldosterone titer.

Aldosterone
In addition to stimulating sodium reabsorption, **aldosterone promotes potassium excretion.** Opposite findings are noted after adrenalectomy. These reciprocal changes in potassium and sodium transport should not be construed as obligatory coupling between sodium reabsorption and potassium secretion. Aldosterone stimulates the basolateral Na–K-ATPase pumps, increases intracellular potassium, raises the gradient between the lumen and cell, and thereby enhances secretion. Aldosterone also increases luminal membrane permeability to potassium so that diffusion into the lumen is more efficient.

Acid-Base Balance
Alterations in systemic acid-base balance affect potassium excretion, primarily through changes in the intracellular concentration of potassium.

1. **Acidosis enhances the movement of potassium out of cells**
2. **Alkalosis enhances the movement of potassium into cells**

Acute alkalosis, either metabolic or respiratory, increases potassium excretion. The opposite is true for acute acidosis. However, potassium excretion with chronic acid-base disturbances is complicated by other factors that tend to blunt or oppose these acute effects (Table 6–1). Only metabolic alkalosis shows consistent effects with resulting large depletions of body potassium.

Delivery of Fluid and Poorly Absorbable Anions to the Distal Tubule
There is an association between rates of distal nephron flow, sodium and poorly absorbable anion excretion, and potassium secretion.

Distal Urine Flow. Restriction of sodium intake results in decreased excretion of both sodium and potassium. Extracellular volume expansion with saline or mannitol solutions and administration of diuretics all enhance the rates of sodium and potassium excretion. Is this effect on potassium excretion related to an increased sodium or fluid delivery to the distal tubule or both? Microperfusion experiments distinguish the effects of these two factors on potassium secretion. When luminal sodium concentration is doubled but tubular flow rate remains constant, potassium secretion does not change. In contrast, a fourfold increase in flow rate without change in tubular sodium concentration doubles potassium secretion. Thus, **the rate of fluid delivery to the distal nephron is a more important determinant of potassium secretion than are the tubular concentration and tubular absorption of sodium.** It is postulated that the lower luminal potassium concentrations associated with higher flow rates permit a larger gradient for diffusion from cell to lumen.

Nonreabsorbed Anions. Under ordinary conditions, the electrochemical gradient between the lumen and cells in the distal nephron favors potassium secretion. The more negative the PD, the greater the secretion. **If the luminal fluid contains a high concentration of nonreabsorbed anions** (sulfate, carbenicillin, ticarcillin, ketoacids) or a greater quantity of bicarbonate than can be reabsorbed proximally (vomiting, respiratory alkalosis, acetazolamide treatment), the negative PD increases, **secretion is enhanced, and increased potassium is lost in the urine.**

TABLE 6–1. ACUTE AND CHRONIC POTASSIUM CHANGES IN URINARY EXCRETION AND STEADY-STATE BODY BALANCE INDUCED BY THE FOUR CARDINAL ACID-BASE DISORDERS

| | Urinary Excretion | | Steady-State Potassium Balance |
	Acute	Chronic	
Respiratory alkalosis	Increased	No change	No change
Metabolic alkalosis	Increased	Increased	Large deficit
Respiratory acidosis	Decreased	Increased	Moderate deficit
Metabolic acidosis	Decreased	Increased	Moderate deficit

POTASSIUM BALANCE

After sodium, potassium is the most prevalent cation in the body and is the major intracellular cation. Total body potassium ranges between 35 and 55 mmol/ kg body weight for men and 30 to 45 mmol/kg for women. This is approximately 3500 mmol in a healthy 70 kg man.

About 70 mmol, or 2% of the total body potassium, is in the ECF at a concentration of 3.5 to 5.0 mmol/L. The remaining 98% is within the cells because of the Na–K-ATPase plasma-membrane pumps that actively transport potassium into most cells. Thus, **cell mass, especially muscle mass, largely determines total body potassium content** (Fig. 6–2).

The concentration of potassium in cell water is between 150 and 160 mmol/L. Because many body functions are highly dependent on the stability of the ionic gradient between ICF and ECF, **derangements in potassium balance are life threatening and require prompt medical intervention to avert cardiac or neuromuscular catastrophe.**

Since 98% of potassium is intracellular and many factors modify the partition between ECF and ICF, **the plasma potassium concentration is only an indirect guide to the status of body stores.** To understand potassium metabolism, it is conceptually useful to divide overall balance into two subsets, **external and internal balance.** External balance is defined as the difference between potassium intake and elimination. Internal balance refers to the distribution between ECF and ICF. It is only when one or the other (or both) of these systems is impaired that marked changes in plasma potassium occur. This is more fully discussed in Chapter 10.

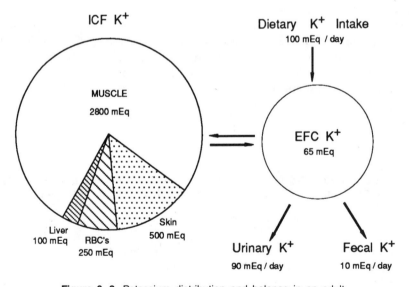

Figure 6–2. Potassium distribution and balance in an adult.

SAMPLE ANSWERS TO STUDY QUESTIONS

1. Based on the concepts presented in this chapter, what fraction of filtered potassium is present at each of the following tubular sites?

| | Diet | | |
Site	Normal(%)	K deficiency (%)	K excess (%)
Beginning of proximal tubule	100	100	100
End of proximal tubule	35	35	35
Early distal tubule	10	10	10
Ureteral urine (fractional excretion)	1–5	1–5	100–200

The following data pertain to Questions 2, 3, and 4. A woman with end-stage renal disease (ESRD) had the following laboratory results.

- 24 hour urine volume = 2.8 L
- $[Creatinine]_u$ = 32 mg/dL
- $[Creatinine]_p$ = 12.5 mg/dL
- $[Potassium]_u$ = 28.6 mmol/L
- $[Potassium]_p$ = 6.0 mmol/L

2. Calculate the fractional excretion of potassium (C_{K^+}/GFR).

$FE_{K^+} = C_{K^+}/GFR$
    $= 1.86$ (or 186%)

3. What do these results indicate about potassium renal transport that is not demonstrable in a healthy subject?

Although data in animals suggest that urinary potassium is derived mainly from distal collecting tubule and duct secretion, net secretion in humans has been difficult to establish because the filtered load is so much larger than the excreted load that most of the potassium is reabsorbed. However, the secretory nature of potassium transport is revealed in advanced renal failure when the excreted load clearly exceeds the filtered load, as in this case.

4. Based on current physiologic concepts, what factors could have produced the potassium fractional excretion data noted in the patient?

All factors that stimulate potassium secretion are present. The elevated plasma potassium concentration would increase intracellular potassium and stimulate aldosterone secretion. Chronic metabolic acidosis probably is present because of retained inorganic acids. Finally, the urine flow rate is high, probably representing an increased fractional excretion of sodium and water.

5. **You are consulted about a patient with persistent hypokalemia (serum K<3 mmol/L). What *single* test would you obtain to confirm renal versus nonrenal causes for this problem?**

   The urine potassium concentration is the best single test. A urinary potassium concentration less than 15 mmol/L would suggest renal reabsorption caused by nonrenal losses. A urinary potassium concentration greater than 15 mmol/L would suggest renal potassium wasting (diuretics, aldosteronism, or a tubular defect) as a primary cause.

6. **Hypokalemia and total body potassium depletion are part of the clinical picture of primary aldosteronism. What two dietary changes would help correct this abnormality? Explain the rationale for your answer.**

   The potassium deficiency and hypokalemia can be corrected partially by supplementing the diet with potassium chloride. However, this often is associated with increased urinary losses, which prevent total correction. Additional correction can be produced by severe dietary sodium restriction. Such restriction reduces the amount of tubular salt and water reaching the distal tubules and thus reduces urinary potassium losses.

Acid-Base Balance: Renal Hydrogen Ion Transport

INTRODUCTION

Acid-base balance is achieved when the hydrogen ion input from the diet and endogenous metabolism and output by all routes of elimination are equal and the extracellular fluid (ECF) hydrogen ion concentration is within physiologic limits:

[H+] 36 to 42 nmol/L, pH 7.38 to 7.44). This chapter considers the sources and routes of elimination of hydrogen ion, focusing on the renal mechanisms for excreting nonvolatile acid.

STUDY QUESTIONS

1. Advanced renal failure is associated with metabolic acidosis from an imbalance between endogenous acid production and reduced renal excretion. What therapeutic plan can you suggest to reduce endogenous acid production in an effort to correct this imbalance?
2. A normal subject in steady-state acid-base balance has a GFR of 120 mL/min and a plasma bicarbonate concentration of 25 mmol/L (or 25 μmol/mL). A 24-hour urine sample had a pH of 5.5 and contained 40 mmol of ammonium and 30 mmol of titratable acid. Calculate
    Bicarbonate reabsorption in μmol/min
    Bicarbonate regenerated from glutamine metabolism in μmol/min
    New bicarbonate generated from TA excretion in μmol/min
    Total renal bicarbonate production in μmol/min *or* mmol/day
3. What is the effect of acetazolamide (a carbonic anhydrase inhibitor) on the following parameters?
    Urine pH
    Ammonium excretion
    Titratable acid excretion
    Systemic acid-base balance
    Questions 4, 5, and 6 pertain to the data in Figure 7–1 illustrating the renal response to chronic acid (ammonium chloride) loading.
4. Why does it take about 10 days to achieve a new steady-state after starting ammonium chloride?
5. Why does the urine pH fall and later rise during ammonium chloride ingestion?
6. What would happen to acid-base balance if renal metabolism of glutamine were impaired?
7. Outline the sequential steps in the development of systemic adaptation to chronic hypercapnia (respiratory acidosis).

HYDROGEN ION BALANCE

Control of hydrogen ion balance differs from regulation of other major electrolytes in three ways.

1. Most of the hydrogen ions excreted are derived from metabolism
2. The hydrogen ions produced exist in two general forms: volatile and non-volatile acids
3. Hydrogen ion balance is achieved by coordinated action of several buffering systems: chemical, pulmonary, hepatic, and renal

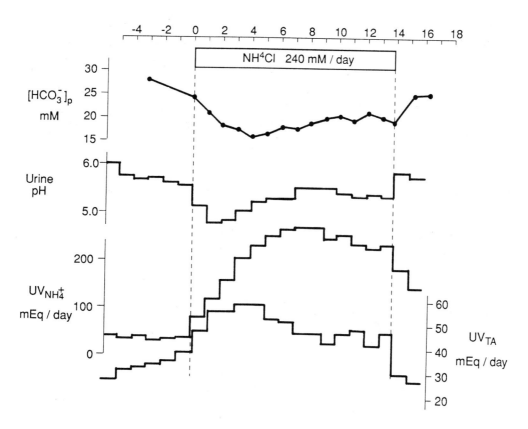

Figure 7–1. The response in a normal subject to acid (NH₄Cl) loading. Changes are plotted in plasma HCO₃ concentration, urine pH, urine ammonium (NH₄), and titratable acid (TA) excretion.

Volatile Acids

Under basal conditions and while ingesting a normal diet, most adults produce about 20,000 mmol of CO_2 daily. This volatile substance, the dehydrated form of carbonic acid (H_2CO_3), is eliminated by the lungs.

Nonvolatile Acid Generation

Oxidation of carbohydrate and triglycerides normally yields only water and CO_2. During illness, formation of lactic acid may occur from carbohydrate metabolism during hypoxic conditions, or ketoacids may be produced from fats in uncontrolled diabetes mellitus.

Most amino acids are metabolized in the liver to glucose or fat and urea. No net acid is generated. Ureagenesis occurs from the combination of bicarbonate and ammonium. The amount of bicarbonate that is produced in amino acid metabolism is large; 500 to 1000 mmol each of HCO_3^- and NH_4^+ result from metabolism of a typical diet. The oxidation of a typical simple amino acid, alanine, is illustrated below.

$$CH_3\text{-}CH\text{-}COO^- + 3O_2 \rightarrow 2CO_2 + HCO_3^- + NH_4^+ + H_2O$$

$$NH_3$$

Nonvolatile acids can be produced from protein catabolism when a neutral amino acid is converted into an anion. This occurs when sulfur- or phosphorus-containing amino acids are converted into sulfuric and phosphoric acid in addition to neutral products. Metabolism of methionine (Met) or cysteine (Cys) is illustrated below.

$$\text{Met or Cys} \rightarrow \text{glucose (or triglyceride)} + \text{urea} + SO_4^{2-} + 2H^+$$

A typical American diet yields about 70 mmol of sulfuric acid and 30 mmol of phosphoric acid daily. Likewise, about 140 mmol of hydrochloric acid are produced by metabolism of cationic amino acids (lysine, arginine, histidine).
Partial buffering of acid comes about when generated hydrogen ions combine with certain anionic metabolites and are further metabolized to neutral end products. For example, **anionic amino acids (glutamate and aspartate) or dietary organic anions (e.g., acetate, lactate, citrate) buffer about 160 mmol of hydrogen ions daily.**

$$\text{Acetate} + H^+ \rightarrow \text{glucose (or triglycerides)} + CO_2$$

About 80 mmol (range, 50 to 100 mmol) of metabolic acid is produced by a typical diet, requiring synthesis of a comparable amount of bicarbonate, a role carried out by the kidneys. However, the role of the kidneys is complementary to hepatic metabolism and the type of diet ingested. Diets low in nitrogen generate a net bicarbonate excess whose excretion in part is accomplished by the kidneys.

Assessment of Hydrogen Ion Balance

It is customary to refer to changes in plasma or blood hydrogen ion concentration, usually expressed as pH (the cologarithm in gram equivalents of hydrogen ions per liter). Such a description implies that the pH in other body fluid compartments correlates closely with plasma pH. Although this seems true for most of the ECF, there are several notable exceptions. For example, pH within cells, cerebrospinal fluid, and on bone surface appears to be influenced in part by factors that may not produce corresponding changes in plasma acidity. Nonetheless, the pH of plasma is measured easily and provides reliable data for the diagnosis and treatment of clinical acid-base disorders.

In addition to the direct measurement of pH, Henderson and Hasselbalch pointed out that complete assessment of acid-base balance also requires measuring the principal buffer system in blood, bicarbonate and carbonic acid. Carbonic acid is the hydrated form of CO_2 and is most conveniently measured as CO_2.

$$pH = 6.1 + \log ([HCO_3^-]/([CO_2])$$

There are other body buffer systems, but they all are in equilibrium with each other (isohydric principle, Fig. 7–2). Evaluation of any one of these buffers, therefore, allows an estimate of changes in all body buffers.

Hydrogen Ion Homeostasis

General Concepts. The continuous production of volatile and nonvolatile acids threatens the stability of the internal environment. The rate of acid production depends on the composition of the diet and the rate of metabolism. Neither factor is under primary control of any hydrogen ion stabilizing system. Thus, pH homeostasis is achieved mainly by adjusting the disposal of the volatile acid, CO_2, and a major buffer, HCO_3^-, so that their ratio remains nearly constant. Elimination of each is controlled by different systems. CO_2 is removed by the lungs. Bicarbonate is excreted by the kidneys or metabolized to CO_2 after buffering hydrogen ion. Nonvolatile acids initially are buffered by body buffers and subsequently are excreted by the kidneys, which simultaneously generate new bicarbonate.

Chemical Buffering of Hydrogen Ions. A primary line of defense against rapid or extreme change in hydrogen ion concentration is **physiochemical buffering.** The presence of chemical buffers in cells and ECF allows the body to titrate quickly large quantities of hydrogen ions without a significant change in the plasma pH. It is important to remember that this type of buffering makes no direct contribution to hydrogen ion removal but only blunts the impact of endogenous acid production on the concentration of hydrogen ion in body fluids.

About 50% of the hydrogen ions entering the ECF are buffered by the carbon dioxide-bicarbonate buffer system.

$$H^+ \text{ input } + HCO_3^- \leftrightarrow H_2CO_3 \leftrightarrow CO_2 + H_2O$$

During this titration of body buffers, bicarbonate is converted to carbonic acid and then to CO_2 and water. As a consequence, the concentration of bicarbonate is reduced. The CO_2 generated is added to the much larger quantity derived from cellular metabolism and is excreted by the lungs.

$$H_nProt \rightleftharpoons Prot^{n-} + H^+ + HPO_4^{2-} \rightleftharpoons H_2PO_4^-$$
$$+$$
$$HCO_3^- \rightleftharpoons H_2CO_3$$

Figure 7–2. The isohydric principle.

Pulmonary Control of Plasma Carbon Dioxide Tension. CO_2 is a volatile acid and normally is controlled at a pressure of about 40 mm Hg by the respiratory system. The large CO_2 production (20,000 mmol/day) from cellular metabolism normally is excreted from the lungs and affects acid-base balance through its influence on carbonic acid concentration. The rate of CO_2 excretion is the product of alveolar ventilation and the alveolar concentration of CO_2. Since CO_2 diffuses readily between the alveoli and alveolar capillaries, the arterial plasma CO_2 tension and alveolar CO_2 tension are identical.

In the steady-state when CO_2 production and excretion are equal, the arterial plasma PCO_2 tension is a reflection of alveolar ventilation. Because alveolar ventilation can be modified rapidly without substantially changing the rate of CO_2 production, the plasma PCO_2 can rise or fall within minutes of a change in the ventilation rate.

Thus, **the normal pulmonary system serves as another line of defense against acid-base perturbations by changing rates of CO_2 excretion.** For example, metabolic acidosis stimulates and alkalosis depresses ventilation. It is obvious that pulmonary dysfunction will cause significant changes in acid-base balance.

Renal Contribution. The kidney excretes hydrogen ions, generates new bicarbonate, and varies its tubular threshold for bicarbonate reabsorption in response to a variety of stimuli described in the next section.

RENAL CONTROL OF PLASMA BICARBONATE

In contrast to the rapid elimination of CO_2 through the lungs, **the renal contribution to HCO_3^- balance is slow. Perturbations require 3 to 5 days for maximal renal response.** The kidneys perform their function in three ways.

1. **reabsorption of the bicarbonate filtered through the glomeruli**
2. **generation of "new" bicarbonate**
3. **regeneration of "old" bicarbonate from glutamine metabolism**

These three processes are totally interrelated and are, in fact, accomplished by a single mechanism, hydrogen ion secretion into tubular fluid and concomitant bicarbonate transport from tubular cells into peritubular blood. Renal dysfunction influences acid-base balance in a variety of ways that may result in either metabolic acidosis or metabolic alkalosis.

Reabsorption of Filtered Bicarbonate

If plasma hydrogen ion concentration is low (metabolic alkalosis with high plasma bicarbonate), plasma pH is adjusted toward normal by reducing the plasma bicarbonate concentration and restoring a normal HCO_3^-/CO_2 ratio. The kidneys can do this in the euvolemic patient with an adequate supply of chloride by limiting reabsorption of filtered bicarbonate, allowing it to be excreted in the urine. In essence, the excretion of a bicarbonate ion in the urine has virtually the same effect on the blood pH as adding a hydrogen ion to the blood. When plasma hydrogen ion concentration is high (acidosis with low plasma bicarbonate), the kidneys reabsorb all the filtered bicarbonate and the tubules generate additional bicarbonate that is contributed to the ECF, thereby returning plasma pH toward normal. The renal addition of bicarbonate to the blood is associated with the excretion of an equal amount of acid in the urine. Thus, **to compensate for alkalosis, the kidneys excrete an alkaline urine and acidify the ECF. In response to acidosis, the kidneys excrete an acid urine**. However, in certain clinical conditions, the kidney may actually contribute to alkalosis by inappropriately excreting an acid urine.

About 4000 mmol of bicarbonate are filtered daily by the glomeruli.

$$
\begin{aligned}
\text{Filtered } HCO_3^-/\text{day} &= GFR \times [HCO_3^-]_p \\
&= 180 \text{ L/day} \times 24 \text{ mmol/L} \\
&= 4320 \text{ mmol/day, or } 4.3 \text{ mol/day}
\end{aligned}
$$

If this bicarbonate were not reabsorbed, it would be equivalent to adding more than 4.3 L of 1 N acid to the body. In the absence of alkalosis, virtually all of the filtered bicarbonate is reabsorbed. Thus, **reabsorption of bicarbonate is normally a conservation process, and none appears in the urine**.

Proximal Tubule. What is the mechanism for bicarbonate reabsorption? Although the tubule is highly permeable to chloride, it is relatively impermeable to bicarbonate. Hence, **bicarbonate reabsorption is an active process**. The accepted hypothesis is the hydrogen ion secretion model (Fig. 7–3).

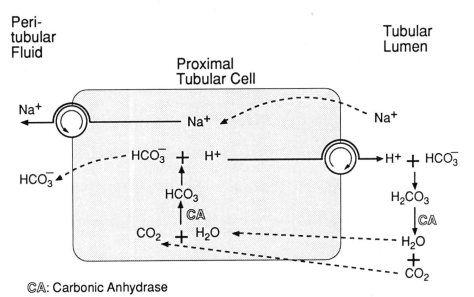

CA: Carbonic Anhydrase

Figure 7–3. Schema of possible processes in bicarbonate reabsorption. In this model, CO_2 is hydrated with the aid of carbonic anhydrase (CA) to form carbonic acid. Secretion of hydrogen ions into tubular lumen occurs probably by an active pump at the luminal border.

When sodium ions that are associated with bicarbonate in the glomerular filtrate are reabsorbed from the luminal fluid by the tubular cell, electroneutrality is maintained by the secretion of an equivalent amount of hydrogen ions into the tubular lumen. When the filtered bicarbonate ions encounter the secreted hydrogen ions, they are converted to carbonic acid, which quickly decomposes to CO_2 and water. The secreted hydrogen ions originate from the intracellular dissociation of carbonic acid, which results from the hydration of CO_2. The rate of this reaction and that in the lumen of the proximal tubule is accelerated by the catalytic influence of the enzyme, carbonic anhydrase. **For each hydrogen ion secreted, a bicarbonate ion also is generated.** These bicarbonate ions generated by the kidneys rather than those originally filtered are the ones conserved by the kidney.

Each segment of the renal tubule concerned with bicarbonate reabsorption and hydrogen ion secretion apparently uses this mechanism. By the end of the proximal tubule, about 80 to 90% of the filtered bicarbonate has been reabsorbed, with a reduction in the tubular fluid pH to 6.5 to 7.0.

Loop of Henle and Distal Nephron. In these segments, bicarbonate reabsorption continues to keep pace with the reabsorption of water or slightly exceeds it, so that the pH of the distal tubular fluid is 6.0 to 6.5. In the collecting duct, the pH falls to that of the final urine.

It is noteworthy that **the hydrogen ion secreted into the lumen for bicarbonate reabsorption is not excreted in the urine. It has combined with bicarbonate in the lumen and been converted rapidly into water and CO_2 and reabsorbed.**

Renal Generation of Bicarbonate and Excretion of Hydrogen Ion

In addition to conserving all of the filtered bicarbonate, the kidneys can generate bicarbonate, so that the quantity of bicarbonate in the renal veins exceeds that which entered the kidneys originally. This alkalinization of the ECF is the renal compensation for the bicarbonate deficit that occurs with buffering of 50 to 100 mmol/day of nonvolatile hydrogen ions. Two basic processes exist: generation of new bicarbonate and production of old bicarbonate from metabolism of glutamine in the renal tubule.

Generation of "New" Bicarbonate. The two renal mechanisms for **producing "new" bicarbonate are tubular secretion of hydrogen ions as "free" (unbuffered) and "titratable" (buffered) acids.** This process is identical to that used in the reabsorption of filtered bicarbonate. The only difference between these two processes is the fate of the secreted hydrogen ion within the tubular lumen. Once filtered bicarbonate is reabsorbed, the secretion of additional hydrogen ions corresponds to the amount of "new" bicarbonate that is generated. These hydrogen ions cannot be recycled through CO_2 and water because bicarbonate ions are no longer present in the tubular fluid. Instead they exist as "free" hydrogen ions or "titratable acids" (TA).

Free, Unbuffered Hydrogen Ions. If 100 mmol of hydrogen ions were excreted as free, unbuffered acid, the final acidity of the urine would be about 100 mmol/L, which corresponds to a urine pH of 1. This degree of acidity in the body is achieved only in gastric fluid. The maximal hydrogen ion concentration attained in the renal tubule is about 0.04 mmol/L, or a pH of 4.4. At this pH, the free hydrogen ion concentration is 1000 times greater in the tubular lumen than in the peritubular plasma. Despite such a gradient, less than 1% of the hydrogen ions secreted by the renal tubules exist in the free state. Most hydrogen ions are excreted in urine with buffers, either nonreabsorbable anions called **titratable acids**, or with secreted ammonia as **ammonium.**

Titratable Acids. When hydrogen ions are secreted into the tubular lumen, causing the pH of the tubular fluid to fall, H^+ binds with the conjugate base (A^-) of a weak acid.

$$H^+ + A^- \leftrightarrow HA$$

Over the usual pH range of urine, phosphate (HPO_4^{2-}) is the major conjugate base that binds secreted H^+. However, when urine pH is 5 or less, creatinine and urate also bind hydrogen ions. This group of conjugate bases is called titratable acids (TA) because they are measured by titrating the urine with sodium hydroxide back to the pH of the blood. Thus, **titratable acids are present only if the urinary pH is less than 7.4.**

For HPO_4^{2-} to act as a conjugate base, it first must be filtered by the glomeruli and then escape reabsorption by the tubules. At the pH of blood, phosphate exists almost entirely in two forms, HPO_4^{2-} (80%) and $H_2PO_4^-$ (20%). If maximum acidification of the urine occurs and the minimal urinary pH of 4.4 is reached, virtually all of the HPO_4^{2-} is converted to $H_2PO_4^-$ (Fig. 7–4). However, about 80% of the

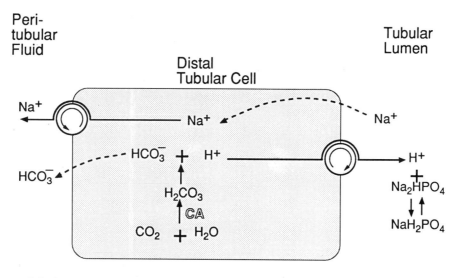

CA: Carbonic Anhydrase

Figure 7–4. Model of titratable acid excretion.

filtered phosphate is reabsorbed and never reaches the distal nephron for this conversion. Furthermore, in the typical diet, only 50% of the ingested phosphate of 30 mmol/day enters the ECF as HPO_4^{2-}, and only a small amount is present to act as a titratable conjugate base. This underscores the quantitative importance of renal glutamine metabolism as the major process for renal regeneration of bicarbonate.

Regeneration of Bicarbonate from Renal Glutamine and Secretion of Ammonium

Ammonium Synthesis and Bicarbonate Generation. During protein metabolism, ammonium and bicarbonate are produced in approximately equal amounts. Ammonium, the conjugate acid of the NH_4^+/NH_3 buffer system, cannot donate hydrogen ions for direct titration of HCO_3^- because it is too weak an acid by a factor of over 1000 (pK$_a$ values are 6.1 for the CO_2/HCO_3^- system and 9.3 for the NH_4^+/NH_3 system). The high pK$_a$ for this buffer system also indicates that NH_4^+ is the predominant molecule at the pH of ECF.

Ammonium in the urine comes from two sources: (1) the filtration of ammonium in renal arterial blood and (2) synthesis of ammonium from glutamine in tubular cells with the catalytic assistance of glutaminase (Fig. 7–5).

Glutamine Metabolism. **The generation of glutamine and urea in the liver and the enzymatic breakdown of glutamine in the kidney are influenced by changes in systemic pH.**

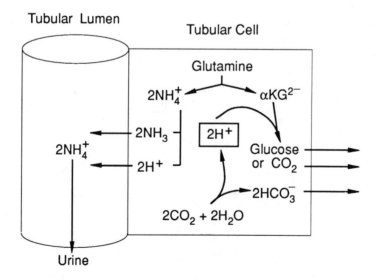

Figure 7–5. Renal hydrogen ion removal associated with ammonium excretion. Hydrogen ions are removed when metabolized in conjunction with alpha-ketoglutarate (α-KG^{2-}), and ammonium secretion occurs secondary to production from glutamine metabolism.

With rising arterial pH, hepatic ureagenesis increases, and glutamine production may stop. Renal metabolism of glutamine diminishes with alkalosis. With systemic acidosis, the opposite hepatic and renal changes occur. When an individual is acidotic for more than a few days, a marked increase in urinary ammonium develops. This increase is, in part, because of increased production of hepatic glutamine, which is transported to the kidney, and increased activity of renal glutaminase.

Most of the ammonium excreted by the kidney is produced by proximal tubule cells, reabsorbed in the thick ascending limb of Henle's loop, concentrated in the medullary interstitium by countercurrent multiplication, and secreted into the urine by transepithelial transport in the collecting ducts.

Quantitation of Renal Acid-Base Function

If acid-base balance is to be maintained, the kidneys must conserve the large load of bicarbonate that is filtered constantly through the glomeruli, excrete 50 to 100 mmol of nonvolatile acid, and add a comparable amount of new bicarbonate to the blood. Thus, tubular acid secretion must be great enough to achieve complete reabsorption of all filtered bicarbonate, plus secreting or removing an additional 50 to 100 mmol of hydrogen ions as TAs and metabolism of glutamine to ammonium and bicarbonate.

The total rate of tubular hydrogen ion secretion is equal to the sum of

Bicarbonate reabsorption + TA excretion + NH_4^+ excretion

Values for a person on a normal diet are approximately

Bicarbonate reabsorption (conservation) = 4300 mmol/day

Titratable acid excretion (HCO_3^- generation) = 30 mmol/day

Ammonium excretion (HCO_3^- regeneration) = 40 mmol/day

Total HCO_3^- (conservation + generation) = 4370 mmol/day

These values emphasize that **the vast majority of secreted hydrogen ions are used for bicarbonate reabsorption**, with only a small amount participating in the generation/regeneration of bicarbonate through TA excretion and renal glutamine metabolism.

Control of Renal Hydrogen Ion Secretion

To this point, the mechanisms for acid secretion by the nephron have been discussed. This section focuses on the factors that stimulate or depress renal excretion of acid.

Systemic Acid-Base Status. If blood pH falls, the renal response is to increase hydrogen ion secretion and produce more bicarbonate through an increase in both TA and ammonium excretion. When blood pH increases and the plasma bicarbonate rises, the kidneys excrete the surplus of bicarbonate as long as the ECF volume is normal. The signal that prompts the kidney to respond appropriately is unknown but may be produced by varying avidity in the sodium-hydrogen ion exchange that normally occurs in the distal nephron.

Changes in Plasma Carbon Dioxide Tension. Chronic hypercapnia (increased plasma PCO_2) increases renal acid secretion and bicarbonate production and elevates the plasma bicarbonate concentration. Thus, patients with chronic pulmonary hypoventilation from any cause (e.g., chronic obstructive pulmonary disease, emphysema) have elevated plasma bicarbonate concentrations. Chronic hypocapnia from hyperventilation (e.g., cirrhosis, brain lesions, some pulmonary lesions, hypoxia from high altitude) reduces renal production of bicarbonate and lowers the plasma bicarbonate concentration.

Potassium Balance. A relationship between potassium and acid-base balance exists (see Chapter 6), but the renal mechanism producing changes in hydrogen ion excretion is unclear. Following a high dietary potassium intake in acute experiments, a reduction of urinary hydrogen ion excretion occurs. On the other hand, severe body potassium deficits of 500 mmol or greater increase urinary hydrogen ion excretion, bicarbonate production, and metabolic alkalosis. Whether these changes in acid excretion have a significant influence on the physiologic regulation of acid-base balance is uncertain.

Changes in the ECF Volume. Although perturbations in the ECF volume modify renal hydrogen ion transport, they do not alter the plasma bicarbonate concentration unless coupled with other factors that produce changes in the plasma electrolytes. For example, severe ECF volume depletion from vomiting and loss of HCl is associated with metabolic alkalosis that is maintained by renal mechanisms until chloride repletion occurs (see Figs. 11–5 and 11–6).

Hormonal Effects. Aldosterone enhances renal sodium-hydrogen ion exchange. Thus, hyperaldosteronism is associated with metabolic alkalosis, whereas hypoaldosteronism may be associated with acidosis. High plasma concentrations of parathyroid hormone decreased bicarbonate reabsorption and are associated with acidosis.

In summary, many ill patients have multiple factors that contribute to an acid-base imbalance. For example, prolonged vomiting may cause severe ECF volume depletion, with circulatory insufficiency and the concomitant development of metabolic alkalosis and organic (lactic) acidosis. The net effect is that systemic pH and urinary acid excretion are quite unpredictable.

SAMPLE ANSWERS TO STUDY QUESTIONS

1. Advanced renal failure is associated with metabolic acidosis from an imbalance between endogenous acid production and reduced renal excretion.

What therapeutic plan can you suggest to reduce endogenous acid production in an effort to correct this imbalance?

Endogenous acid production depends principally on metabolism of protein from dietary and body tissue turnover (catabolism). By reducing the amount of protein metabolism and providing a high biologic quality (mainly essential amino acids) of dietary protein, a reduced production of inorganic (sulfuric and phosphoric) acids occurs. By treating or preventing catabolism (treat infections, avoid antimetabolites and cytotoxic or catabolic drugs), a decrease in production of both inorganic and organic acids will occur. Short courses of anabolic drugs (androgens) also may be helpful.

2. **A normal subject in steady-state acid-base balance has a GFR of 120 mL/min and a plasma bicarbonate concentration of 25 mmol/L (or 25 μmol/mL). A 24-hour urine sample had a pH of 5.5 and contained 40 mmol of ammonium and 30 mmol of titratable acid. Calculate**

Bicarbonate reabsorption (equals filtered load)

$$\text{GFR} \times [\text{HCO}_3]_p = 120 \text{ mL/min} \times 25 \text{ } \mu\text{mol/mL} = 3000 \text{ } \mu\text{mol/min}$$

Bicarbonate regenerated from glutamine metabolism (equals ammonium excretion)

$$\frac{40,000 \text{ } \mu\text{mol/day}}{1440 \text{ min/day}} = 28 \text{ } \mu\text{mol/min}$$

New bicarbonate generated from TA excretion

$$\frac{30,000 \text{ } \mu\text{mol/day}}{1440 \text{ min/day}} = 21 \text{ } \mu\text{mol/min}$$

Total renal bicarbonate production = 3049 μmol/min, or 4391 mmol/day

3. **What is the effect of acetazolamide (a carbonic anhydrase inhibitor) on the following parameters?**
   Urine pH
   Ammonium excretion
   Titratable acid excretion
   Systemic acid-base balance

Acetazolamide inhibits carbonic anhydrase in the renal tubular cell and reduces hydrogen ion secretion and intracellular bicarbonate production. Thus, bicarbonate reabsorption in the proximal tubule and generation from all cells throughout the tubule are impaired. Expected changes resulting from this inhibition are as follows.

Urine pH: rises because of an increase in urine bicarbonate without a concomitant increase in P_{CO_2}.

Ammonium excretion: the amount appearing in the urine is indirectly proportional to the urine pH. Thus, as urine pH rises, less glutamine is metabolized and ammonium excretion is reduced.

Titratable acid excretion: the reduced secretion of hydrogen ions limits the amount that will be buffered, and excretion falls.

Systemic acid-base balance: the loss of filtered bicarbonate and reduction of bicarbonate generation by the kidney produces a systemic metabolic acidosis with a decrease in pH of the blood.

Questions 4,5, and 6 pertain to the data in Figure 7–6 illustrating the renal response to chronic acid (ammonium chloride) loading.

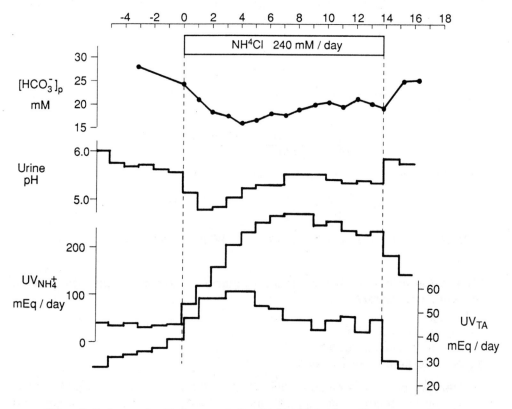

Figure 7–6. A normal subject responds to acid (NH_4Cl) loading. Changes are plotted in plasma HCO_3^- concentration and parameters of uring acid excretion.

4. Why does it take about 10 days to achieve a new steady-state after starting ammonium chloride?

The ingestion of a large daily ammonium chloride load increases the intake of inorganic acid and ammonia (NH_3–HCl) that must be metabolized (NH_3) or excreted (HCl). The acid initially is buffered, as shown by the fall in plasma bicarbonate. There is a concomitant rise in urinary hydrogen ions as unbuffered ions (fall in urine pH). There is also a rise in renal bicarbonate production from both TA (largely from the fall in urinary pH) and glutamine metabolism (exhibited as a rise in ammonium excretion). This slow but progressive increase in renal bicarbonate production ameliorates the prior fall in the plasma bicarbonate. However, correction is slow, particularly for increased hepatic synthesis of glutamine, and requires about 10 days to reach its maximal effect.

5. Why does the urine pH fall and later rise during ammonium chloride ingestion?

The initial fall in urine pH represents an increase in unbuffered hydrogen ions before a significant increase in urinary buffers (TA and ammonium) has occurred. As TA increases, the unbuffered hydrogen ions diminish and urine pH rises.

6. What would happen to acid-base balance if renal metabolism of glutamine were impaired?

The increase in glutamine synthesis and renal degradation noted in this study (i.e., increased urinary ammonium excretion) was a major source of bicarbonate regeneration after ammonium chloride loading. A defect in glutamine metabolism would reduce this source of bicarbonate production and thus prevent correction of the systemic metabolic acidosis.

7. Outline the sequential steps in the development of systemic adaptation to chronic hypercapnia (respiratory acidosis).

When CO_2 is retained, as during alveolar hypoventilation from any cause, the Pco_2 rises. As the CO_2 is hydrated, H^+ and HCO_3^- are produced. This H^+ must be buffered by nonbicarbonate buffers (e.g., proteins, organic phosphates). Since the primary disturbance is respiratory, the adaptive response will be renal, and it takes days to come to completion. The renal response involves increased reabsorption of bicarbonate secondary to the elevated plasma Pco_2 and increased bicarbonate production from TA and glutamine metabolism secondary to acidosis. This is one instance in which the plasma bicarbonate is elevated in the presence of systemic acidosis.

Body Fluids and Compartments

INTRODUCTION

The internal environment regulated by the kidneys is a water solution containing various solutes. This solution is distributed in several anatomic compartments. This chapter describes the size and the distinctive composition of these compartments, as well as critical factors that maintain differences between the compartments.

STUDY OBJECTIVES

1. Identify the body fluid compartments.
2. Characterize the body fluid compartments according to:
   a. Size
   b. Composition

3. Understand the terms:
    a. Osmolarity
    b. Osmolar forces
    c. Oncotic pressure
4. Know the relationship between Na^+ content and extracellular volume (ECV).
5. Understand the relationship between osmolarity and intracellular volume (ICV).
6. Understand the Starling forces.
7. Recognize major causes of edema.
8. Define tonicity (hyper-, hypo-, iso-).

Rather than providing specific answers to these objectives, the study problems at the end of the chapter attempt to clarify them.

COMPARTMENTS

Total Body Water
The water content of humans varies in relation to the amount of fat present. Fat contains very little water. Indeed, carcass analysis reveals a **direct relationship between lean body mass (LBM) and total body water (TBW).**

$$\text{LBM} = \frac{\text{TBW}}{0.732}$$

Table 8–1 illustrates weight–body water relationships based on build and sex. Women have a greater percentage of body fat. **For practical purposes, we can assume that all adults have 60% of body weight as water. Thus, a 70 kg man has a 42 L TBW.**

Body Water Compartments
Various membranes separate body water into compartments (Fig. 8–1). The **TBW is distributed between two major compartments, the intracellular and the extracellular. The intracellular compartment is larger,** comprising nearly two thirds of the TBW. **The smaller extracellular compartment has two major subdivisions, the plasma and interstitial subdivisions, comprising about 4% and 15% of the body weight, respectively.** Lymph, constituting 2 to 3% of the body weight, is included in the interstitial volume.

    The transcellular compartment is a third, usually minor, subdivision of the extracellular space. It is defined by being separated by a layer of epithelium. The transcellular compartment includes (1) cerebrospinal, (2) intraocular, (3) pleural, (4)

TABLE 8–1. BODY WATER EXPRESSED AS A PERCENTAGE OF BODY WEIGHT

Build	Infant	Adult Male	Adult Female
Thin	80	65	55
Average	70	60	50
Obese	65	55	45

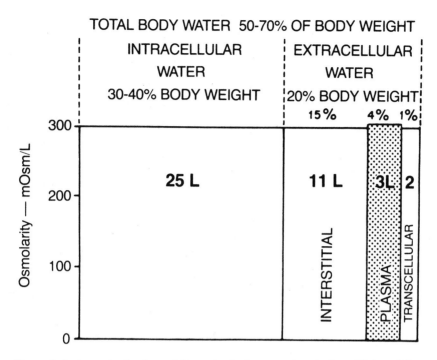

Figure 8–1. Approximate sizes of the major body compartments for a 70 kg adult.

peritoneal, and (5) synovial fluids as well as digestive secretions. Normally only 1% of body weight, the transcellular compartment under certain pathologic conditions (e.g., pleural effusions, ascites) may become a large portion of the total extracellular fluid.

When the transcellular compartment is unusually large, it often is referred to as a third space because fluid in this compartment is not readily exchangeable with the rest of the extracellular fluid (ECF).

The rapid rate of fluid shift between the interstitial and plasma compartments of the extracellular fluid is protective, allowing acute changes in the plasma volume to be distributed quickly throughout the ECF. Fluid shifts between the intracellular and extracellular compartments result from osmolar changes and do not assist in defending plasma volume.

Chemical Composition

Although the types of solutes in both the intracellular and extracellular compartments are similar, their concentrations are strikingly different (Fig. 8–2). Intracellular fluid (ICF) contains large quantities of potassium, phosphate, magnesium, and protein, with small amounts of sodium, calcium, chloride, and bicarbonate.

In ECF, the distribution is reversed. The principal electrolytes in the ECF are sodium, calcium, chloride, and bicarbonate. These differences between ECF and ICF are maintained by active cellular transport processes.

Despite the different distributions of the various substances in the ECF and ICF, the total chemical reactivity of the cations is equal to that of the anions

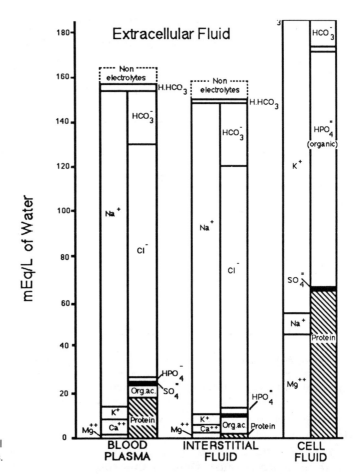

Figure 8–2. The chemical composition of body fluids.

within each compartment. In each compartment, the total positive charges are balanced by an equivalent number of negative charges. **This balance of positive and negative charges is called electrical neutrality.**

Explanation for Compositional Differences

Gibbs-Donnan Equilibrium. **Most capillaries are permeable to small ions and molecules but are nearly impermeable to plasma proteins and larger particles.** Hence, the interstitial space generally contains less than 10 g/L of protein. This low value is contrasted with that of plasma, which contains 70 g/L of protein. Because capillaries are highly permeable to water and small ions, one might expect a uniform electrolyte distribution between plasma and interstitial fluid. However, such is not the case.

The presence of a higher concentration of negatively charged protein in the plasma causes an asymmetrical distribution of diffusible extracellular ions (mainly sodium, chloride, and bicarbonate) between plasma and interstitial fluid. This is commonly referred to as the Gibbs-Donnan equilibrium.

Permeability. The difference in osmolarity between the two compartments is not only because of contained protein but also because the sum of the diffusible ions on the side containing the protein is greater than the sum of those ions on the other side. **The total difference in osmotic pressure that is due to the Gibbs-Donnan effect is known as oncotic pressure.** Albumin accounts for 65% of the oncotic pressure in plasma.

The differences between interstitial fluid and ICF composition are related to selective permeabilities of cellular membranes not only for proteins but also for certain other ions, such as the organic phosphates. In addition, these membranes exhibit active transport mechanisms that maintain high intracellular potassium concentrations and largely exclude sodium. Since most of the intracellular anions are barred from the interstitial fluid by the cell membrane, the Gibbs-Donnan effect also applies. Finally, there is a high probability that certain ions bind to intracellular proteins and phosphates.

Thus, the **large compositional differences between ICF and ECF result from four factors.**

1. **Selective permeabilities of cellular membranes**
2. **Metabolic pumps**
3. **Gibbs-Donnan forces**
4. **Ion binding**

OSMOLAR COMPOSITION AND ONCOTIC PRESSURE

Total solute concentration is expressed in terms of osmolarity. Normal osmolar concentration of body fluids is 290 ± 10 milliosmols/liter (mOsm/L). The number of milliosmols is determined by the number of particles in a solution, whether the particles are molecules or ions. Each particle has a unit value of 1, regardless of its size or charge. If a substance ionizes, each ion contributes to the osmolarity the same amount as one nonionizable molecule. For example, 1 mmol of glucose, a nonionizable molecular substance, in 1 L of water has an osmolar concentration of 1 mOsm/L. On the other hand, 1 mmol of calcium chloride ($CaCl_2$) in 1 L of water forms 3 ions, 1 calcium and 2 chlorides, and has an osmolar concentration of 3 mOsm/L.

Sodium and its attendant anions (mainly chloride and bicarbonate) constitute 90 to 95% of the osmotically active solutes in the ECF (Fig. 8–2). Remember that osmolarity must be distinguished from electrical equivalency. In osmolarity, the charge of particles is irrelevant; rather it is the number of particles that counts.

It has been shown by a number of experimental techniques that the **osmolarity of interstitial fluid is equal to that of ICF.** This observation does not conflict with the differences shown in Figure 8–2. If the interstitial and intracellular concentrations were expressed as millimoles per liter of water and the appropriate dissociation constants were applied to each compound, the calculated osmolarities in both compartments would be comparable, as shown in Figure 8–1.

In contrast, the **osmolarity of plasma is slightly higher than that of interstitial fluid and ICF.** This difference **is due to the high protein content of plasma** (70 g/L). Although relatively small amounts of protein leak into the interstitium (10 g/ L), permeability is so small that the capillary wall behaves as a **semipermeable membrane,** limiting the distribution of plasma proteins. Hence, a protein osmotic pressure develops that tends to pull fluid into the capillaries. This protein osmotic pressure is opposed by hydrostatic pressure gradients generated by the heart, allowing the osmotic pressure differences to persist in equilibrium. **For practical purposes, the body compartments can be considered osmotically equal.**

MAINTENANCE OF COMPARTMENT SIZE

Importance of Total Solute Content

Consider the following equation as it applies to body fluid compartments.

$$\text{Solute concentration (mOsm/L)} = \frac{\text{total solutes}}{\text{volume}}$$

The ICF normally has a fixed total solute content maintained by active transport. Therefore, water movement alters cell size (and hence ICF volume). Thus, changes in compartment osmolarity reflect changes in ICF volume. Since ECF and ICF osmolarity are equal (Fig. 8–1), plasma osmolarity reflects ICF size. In contrast to ICF, the ECF may have changes in total solute and/or solute concentration. Therefore, the ECF volume cannot be inferred from the osmolarity measurement.

Let us examine how changes in solute content affect the ECF. The effects of changes in osmolarity on ECF are discussed later. Recall that sodium and its attendant anions constitute 90 to 95% of the osmotically active particles in the ECF. The effect of adding 5 L of an isosmolar solution of NaCl (0.9% solution contains about 150 mEq/L) is shown in Figure 8–3. Since sodium is excluded from cells, it remains in the extracellular compartment. Chloride will remain with sodium to maintain electrical neutrality. Thus, **when a sodium solution is given, the solute is added entirely to the extracellular volume.** Because osmotic equilibrium also must be maintained, the water given with the saline also will remain outside the cells. **Therefore, clinical manifestations of saline excess result from extracellular volume overload. This can cause edema, hypertension, pulmonary congestion, or ascites.**

Regulation of Plasma and Interstitial Volumes

The distribution of ECF between the plasma and interstitial spaces is regulated at the level of the capillaries and lymphatics (Fig. 8–4). **Fluid movement is governed by Starling forces.** This relationship is depicted in the following formula.

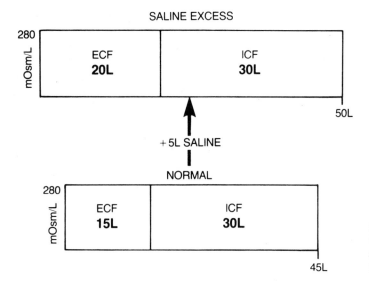

Figure 8–3. The effect of infusing 5 L of an isosmolar solution of NaCl (saline) on the ECF volume.

$$JF = Kj [(Pc + t) - (Pt + c)]$$

Outward   Inward

forces   forces

where JF = filtration flow, Kj = filtration coefficient, Pc = capillary hydraulic pressure: arterial, 32 mmHg; venous, 15 mmHg, t = tissue oncotic pressure, 2 mmHg, Pt = tissue hydraulic pressure, 2 mmHg, c = capillary oncotic pressure, 25 mmHg.

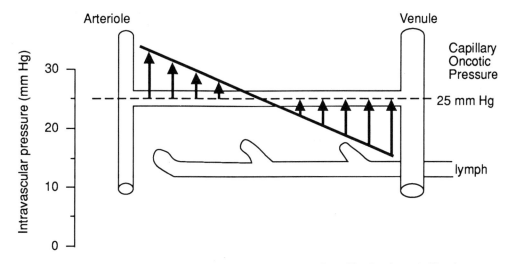

Figure 8–4. Diagram of fluid shifts along an average capillary (Starling forces). Filtration flow depicted by vertical arrows.

Ninety percent of filtered fluid returns to the capillary at more distal portions of the capillary, where hydraulic pressure is lower and oncotic pressure higher because of prior movement of fluid out of the capillary. Ten percent of the fluid normally is returned to the circulation by the lymphatics.

The Starling hypothesis suggests four possible reasons for the appearance of edema (ECF excess), as noted in Table 8–2.

Regulation of Intracellular Volume

Active Transport and Simple Diffusion. Cells have a high oncotic pressure and are freely permeable. Why do they not swell with water and burst? This does not occur because the distribution of solutes between the ICF and the interstitial compartment is not governed simply by the Gibbs-Donnan forces. Rather, **intracellular solutes are carefully controlled by active transport processes.** Thus, sodium chloride outside the cell and potassium and organic solutes inside the cell represent the major effective solutes that determine the osmolarity of ECF and ICF, respectively.

Solutes such as urea that cross cellular membranes by simple diffusion have no net effect on the cell volume, since they eventually reach the same concentrations in both ICF and ECF. **Only nonpenetrating solutes** (e.g., sodium chloride, glucose, mannitol) **alter cell volume.** They do so by producing a change in the ECF osmolarity, which comes into equilibrium by movement of water out of the ICF.

Tonicity of Solutions: Isotonic, Hypotonic, Hypertonic. A simple example at this point may be useful. Red blood cells removed from the body and placed in solutions containing different concentrations of sodium chloride change their volume according to the osmolarity of these solutions. If the osmolarity of the solution in which the cells are suspended is lower than the osmolarity of the cells, water diffuses into the cells, causing them to swell. The cells shrink if the osmolarity of the solution outside is greater than that inside the cell. By comparing the volume of the cell as it exists in the body with its volume in different sodium chloride solutions, the salt concentration that is associated with no change in the

TABLE 8–2. CLINICAL DISTURBANCES OF THE MICROCIRCULATION CAUSING EDEMA

Force Affected	Example and Cause
Increased capillary hydraulic pressure	Increased venous resistance due to thrombophlebitis or heart failure
Decreased plasma oncotic pressure	Hypoalbuminemia due to starvation, nephrotic syndrome, or liver failure
Increased tissue oncotic pressure	Increased capillary permeability due to burns, inflammation, lymphatic blockage
Increased tissue hydraulic pressure due to decreased lymphatic flow	Lymphatic blockage due to neoplasms or surgery

cell volume must have the same concentration of nonpenetrating particles as the red cell. Such a solution is said to be isotonic to those cells.

An **isotonic solution is any solution in which the cell volume remains the same as when surrounded by body fluids. Solutions in which the cells swell are called hypotonic, and solutions in which the cells shrink are called hypertonic solutions.** In this example, a solution of 300 mOsm/L of sodium chloride was found to be isotonic for human red cells. Any other solution containing 300 mOsm/L of **nonpenetrating** solutes also is isotonic. Urea at 300 mOsm/L crosses the red cell membrane along with water, causing the cell to swell. Urea is, therefore, isosmotic but hypotonic.

Infusion of Hypotonic and Hypertonic Solutions. The normal fluid status is depicted in the middle of Figure 8–5, and the changes that occur following infusion of 5% glucose solution are depicted at the top. Although the 5% glucose solution is isosmolar to plasma, glucose is metabolized rapidly, leaving behind 3 L of solute-free water. This water distributes between the ECF and ICF in proportion to their original volumes; that is, 2 L of water enter the ICF, and 1 L remains in the ECF. With this increase in total body water, the osmolarity of the body fluids

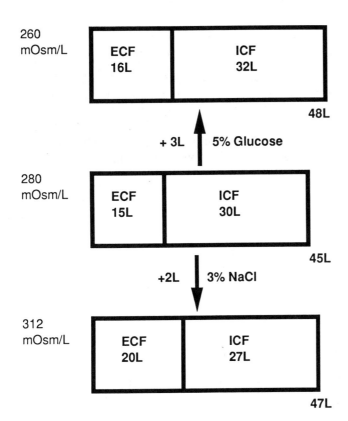

Figure 8–5. Infusion of water (5% glucose) and hypertonic saline (3% NaCl).

decreases from 280 to 260 mOsm/L. **Hence, as osmolarity falls, both the ECF volume and ICF volume increase.**

In the lower part of Figure 8–5, 2 L of a 3% solution of NaCl (1026 mOsm/L) are infused. Because the intracellular compartment is essentially impermeable to the NaCl solution the infused solution remains in the extracellular compartment, and, in addition, an increase in osmolarity occurs, drawing water from the ICF. At equilibrium, the total body osmolarity is increased from 280 to 312 mOsm/L, the ICF volume has decreased by 3 L, and the ECF volume has increased by 5 L. Thus, **changes in body osmolarity often affect both ICF and ECF volumes conversely.** ICF volume, however, changes in the opposite direction from osmolarity. When osmolarity rises, water content is being lost, and ICF volume drops. When osmolarity decreases, water is accumulating, and ICF volume rises.

STUDY PROBLEMS

Problem 1. A 4-year-old African boy developed a potbelly, red hair, and swollen legs. He was weak and small for his age. The concentration of serum albumin was very low (1.5 g/dL). His chief source of food since weaning has been manioc root, which is rich in starch and poor in protein. He was diagnosed as having kwashiorkor.

    1. Explain the pathogenesis of his swollen abdomen and legs.
    2. What are the physiologic factors involved in the development of his edema?

Problem 2. By adding various types of solutions to whole blood and noting the effect of various parameters, a better understanding of the factors influencing the maintenance of body compartments is obtained. In the following experiment, assume that the red cells represent the intracellular compartment, and the plasma represents the extracellular compartment. Relate the differences noted to what you have just learned about factors that change the volumes of body fluid compartments.

Experiment 1.

Changes in Whole Blood Diluted with Water

Sample	Water mL	Blood mL	Hct %	Hgb g/dL	Plasma K	Na mEq/L
0	0	4	45.2	15.3	3.8	140
1	0.2	4	44.4	14.2	3.7	136
2	0.4	4	44.3	13.4	3.5	130
3	0.6	4	44.0	12.7	3.5	120
4	0.8	4	44.0	12.3	3.2	113
5	1.0	4	44.0	11.3	2.5	103

    3. What happened to the red cell volume and the plasma volume?

4. Why did the hematocrit (Hct) remain constant and the hemoglobin (Hgb) concentration fall?

Experiment 2. When equal volumes of distilled water, isosmolar solutions of urea and sodium chloride were added to whole blood, the following results were obtained:

		Blood		Plasma	
		Hct	Hgb	K	Na
Fluid Added		**%**	**g/dL**	**mEq/L**	
Water	Control	45.2	15.3	3.7	140
	Test	44.0	11.3	2.5	103
Isosmolar	Control	44.1	14.6	4.0	138
urea	Test	43.5	11.3	3.1	100
Isosmolar	Control	46.0	13.3	4.0	144
NaCl	Test	33.5	10.6	3.0	146

5. Discuss these results.
6. If isosmolar glucose instead of isosmolar urea had been added, what would have occurred? (Would similar results be expected when isosmolar glucose is given intravenously to humans?)

Problem 3. A patient without kidney function is given 3 L of fluid intravenously in a period of a few hours.

7. Assuming an initial body weight of 70 kg, what will be his final weight?
8. During the interval in question, the patient's plasma osmolarity did not change. Calculate the change in his intracellular and extracellular spaces.
9. What kind of fluid did the patient receive?

Another functionally anephric patient was given 3 L of isotonic saline and 3 L of 5% dextrose in water. His initial serum sodium was 140 mEq/L but fell to 130 mEq/L after the fluid infusions.

10. Assuming no fluid or electrolyte losses occurred during the period of infusion and an initial normal fluid balance, calculate the change in the size of the intracellular and extracellular compartments.
11. If his initial weight was 70 kg, what would his final weight be?
12. In the absence of changes in nonhydrous tissue mass, changes in body weight are caused by changes in the ECF and ICF volumes, that is

$$\Delta \text{ Body weight } = \Delta \text{ ECF } + \Delta \text{ ICF}$$

Use the change in serum sodium concentration and the equation to calculate changes in this patient's ECF and ICF volumes, again assuming his initial weight is 70 kg.

ANSWERS TO STUDY PROBLEMS

Problem 1.
1. Reduced plasma osmotic pressure is the only abnormality in this child.

Normal serum albumin concentration = 5 g/dL
5 g/dL = 28 mm Hg osmotic pressure
Osmotic pressure (x) in the kwashiorkor patient

$$\frac{5 \text{ g/dL}}{28 \text{ mm Hg}} = \frac{1.5 \text{ g/dL}}{x}, \text{ so } x = 8.4 \text{ mm Hg}$$

Change in osmotic pressure = 28 − 8.4 = 19.6 mm Hg

2. Filtration and reabsorption across capillaries results from the balance among capillary and tissue hydrostatic pressures and plasma and interstitial fluid protein concentrations. It can be expressed as follows.

F = k[(Pc − Pi) − (c − i)] where F = filtration (−F = reabsorption), k = filtration constant, Pc = capillary hydrostatic pressure, Pi = interstitial hydrostatic pressure, πc = plasma colloid osmotic pressure, πi = interstitial colloid osmotic pressure

Plasma colloid osmotic pressure is decreased so that the balance across the capillaries is thrown off in favor of filtration. Filtration continues until the low capillary colloid osmotic pressure is balanced by a high interstitial hydrostatic pressure caused by the increased volume. This edema fluid is the cause for the swollen abdomen and legs.

3. What happened to the red cell volume? The plasma volume?

It is assumed that the osmolarity in plasma and in body cells is the same. In the experiment, the addition of increasing amounts of distilled (solute-free) water to a constant amount of whole blood produced an increase in the total amount of water present. Because the osmolarity between plasma and red cells is the same, the water distributes proportionately between these two compartments, and the plasma and red cell volume both are increased.

4. Why did the hematocrit remain constant? Why did the hemoglobin concentration fall?

The hematocrit is, by definition, the relative volume occupied by the red cells in proportion to the amount of total blood measured. In health, the hematocrit is 45 ± 5%. The addition of solute-free water would be expected to dilute all solutes present in the blood, but the hematocrit did not significantly change despite an increasing volume of water. This constancy of the hematocrit is due to an increase in red cell volume, which is proportional to the increase in plasma volume. Thus, the red cells swell in proportion to the solute-free water added, and the hematocrit remains constant.

In contrast to the hematocrit, the hemoglobin falls because it represents the concentration of a certain solute (Hgb) in relationship to the solvent (water) present. Thus, a fixed amount of hemoglobin is present clinically and is diluted by addition of water, as reflected by a fall in its concentration. This is also true for the concentration of plasma sodium (and chloride also if it had been measured).

Although the concentration of plasma potassium fell in this experiment, it does not change significantly with water excess clinically. The largest reservoir of potassium is present intracellularly, and the plasma concentration is maintained by active transport mechanisms.

5. **Discuss the results of experiment 2.**

Hematocrit. The water present in the isosmolar urea solution has distributed itself equally between the plasma and the red cell volume. The result is similar to that seen with distilled water because urea penetrates cells easily. The urea was not confined to the plasma volume but distributed itself, as did the water, equally between the plasma and the red cell volume, and the hematocrit did not change. On the other hand, the addition of an isosmolar sodium chloride solution produced a distinct fall in the hematocrit. Because active red cell transport mechanisms maintained the sodium outside of the cell, there was no change in red cell volume but a marked increase in the plasma volume and, thus, a decrease in the hematocrit.

Plasma sodium concentration. The plasma concentration fell as it was diluted by sodium-free solutions but not with the isosmolar sodium chloride solution. This is similar to clinical situations in which excessive sodium-free fluid is retained.

Hemoglobin and potassium. The amount of each of these solutes was constant in the experiment, and the addition of solutions without these solutes led to a decrease in their concentration. Clinically, it is common in states of excess water, isosmolar urea, and saline infusions to see a fall in the hemoglobin. It is unusual for the serum potassium concentration to be significantly changed clinically in any of the conditions noted.

6. **If isosmolar glucose instead of isosmolar urea had been added, would the results have been any different?**

In the test tube experiment, little glucose would have been transported into the cell, and thus, it would have mimicked the isosmolar sodium chloride experiment by reducing the hematocrit. However, other changes would have been similar to the distilled water or isosmolar urea study. The experimental situation differs significantly from the clinical situation because glucose transport into most body cells is rapid. Thus, clinically, isosmolar glucose mimics the addition of distilled water to blood, and administering glucose is similar to administering solute-free water to the body. On the other hand, the clinical administration of isosmolar mannitol (a hexose-like sugar that is not transported into cells or metabolized) would mimic the test tube study with isosmolar glucose, and a fall in hematocrit and plasma sodium would be seen.

7. **Assuming an initial body weight of 70 kg, what will be the patient's final weight?**

3 L = 3 kg
Therefore
Final weight = 70 kg + 3 kg = 73 kg

8. **Calculate the change in the size of the intracellular and extracellular spaces.**

The change in the size of these spaces depends on the type of fluid given. These permutations are considered, then, in the next problem (9).

9. **What kind of fluid did the patient receive?**

The lack of significant change in the plasma osmolarity means that an isosmolar solution was given. The change in ECF and ICF is variable and dependent on the type of isosmolar solution. If we also find that the plasma sodium concentration does not change, we can assume that an isosmolar solution of a sodium salt, for example, NaCl or $NaHCO_3$, was used. In this instance, all of the administered solution would remain in the ECF, and it would be expanded by 3 L.

Another possibility might be that the plasma sodium concentration fell. This would reflect the administration of an isosmolar solution that does not contain sodium. If the solute in question is unable to penetrate cells readily, it would remain in the ECF and cause it to expand by 3 L at the same time the plasma sodium concentration is decreasing due to dilution by a nonsodium-containing solution. On the other hand, if the isosmolar solution contains a penetrating solute, such as urea, the solution will distribute into the total body water proportionate to the size of each compartment. Hence, ICF will increase by approximately 2 L and ECF by 1 L in this instance.

10. **Calculate the change in the size of the intracellular and extracellular compartments.**

The isotonic solution of saline (NaCl) would remain in the ECF, increasing the volume by 3 L. However, the 5% dextrose solution is equivalent to 3 L of distilled water, since the glucose is rapidly metabolized. Thus, this solution is distributed throughout the total body water proportionate to compartment size; that is, 2 L enters the ICF and 1 L remains in the ECF. The end result is

Space	Saline		Water	Total	
ECF	3L	+	1L	=	4L
ICF	0	+	2L	=	2L

11. What is the final weight?

70 kg + 6 L (kg) = 76 kg

12. Calculate changes in ECF and ICF volumes.

In order to make this calculation, it must be recalled that a change in ICF volume occurs only when the osmolarity changes. In this instance, the decrease in the serum sodium to 130 mEq/L reflects a decrease in osmolarity and an increase in the ICF volume from the addition of solute-free fluid (5% dextrose in water—the dextrose is metabolized to CO_2). The change in serum sodium concentration is proportional to the change in intracellular volume.

$$\text{Body weight} = \text{ECF} + \text{ICF}$$
$$+6L \text{ (kg)} = \text{ECF} + \frac{140 - 130(0.4 \times 70 \text{ kg})}{140}$$

(Hint: 0.4 (or 40%) represents the proportion of the body weight that is ICF volume.)

$$+6L = \text{ECF} + 2L$$
$$4L = \text{ECF}$$

Saline and Water

Nonfluid Mass
Treatment Guidelines
STUDY CASES
ANSWERS TO STUDY CASES

INTRODUCTION

Disturbances of water and electrolyte balance may occur when a patient becomes seriously ill from any cause. Whenever the heart, kidneys, liver, or lungs are diseased or malfunctioning, fluid imbalance is particularly prone to develop since these are the prime regulators of the internal environment. Obviously, if large amounts of body fluid are lost through vomiting and diarrhea, the disturbance can be acute, severe, and even fatal.

In this chapter, we consider disorders of water balance and sodium balance.

Terminology

The word dehydration causes confusion because it commonly is used to describe various combinations of disorders of sodium and water balance. **It is not used in this chapter.** In its place, specific terms, such as "saline excess" and "water depletion," are used. These terms accurately delineate the disorder and imply corrective therapy.

STUDY OBJECTIVES

To understand the

1. Causes
2. Diagnosis
3. Management

of the following fluid balance disorders

1. Water excess
2. Water depletion
3. Saline excess
4. Saline depletion

WATER DISORDERS

Physiology

Water Content. **The water content of cells determines cell volume and is estimated by extracellular osmolarity.** Because the osmotically active particles within cells are retained there, cell volume is determined by water content. Since water moves freely across cell walls, it equilibrates between the extracellular and intracellular compartments so that osmolarity (a measure of the total particles dissolved in a fixed volume of water) is the same in both compartments. Measurement of osmolarity in the blood, a readily accessible portion of the extracellular volume (ECV), then, reflects intracellular volume (ICV).

It must be remembered, however, that **osmolarity correlates inversely with cell volume.** As water is added to the system, the osmolarity falls. As water is lost from the system osmolarity rises. Therefore, **a high serum osmolarity means water depletion (ICV depletion), and a low serum osmolarity means water excess (ICV excess).**

Serum Sodium Concentration. **Serum sodium concentration reflects osmolarity.** Since sodium and its accompanying anions make up almost 95% of the osmolarity of the ECF, sodium concentration almost always correlates closely with osmolarity. **Hyponatremia (low serum sodium) usually is diagnostic of water excess, whereas hypernatremia implies water depletion.**

Artifacts. **Occasionally the serum sodium can be misleading. Hyperglycemia is the most common clinical situation in which this occurs.** Like sodium, glucose is distributed in the extracellular space. Hence, when the blood glucose becomes acutely elevated, extracellular osmolarity increases, and water moves from the cells to the extracellular space, diluting the serum sodium level. To correct for this dilution, **add 2.0 mEq/L to the observed serum sodium level for every 100 mg/dL that the blood sugar is elevated.** (This is a close approximation that simplifies calculations.) This corrected sodium represents the value that would be found if the glucose were not elevated and more accurately reflects the osmolarity than true serum sodium.

Example: A patient with a diabetic ketoacidosis has a serum sodium of 120 mEq/L and a blood glucose of 1100 mg/dL. The corrected serum sodium level would be 140 mEq/L. This result is derived from the 1000 mg% the glucose is elevated, multiplied by 2 mEq for every 100 mg% of elevation.

Marked elevation in BUN also increases body osmolarity. Here no correction is necessary because urea is distributed throughout the total body water, and its presence does not draw water out of cells to change cell volume or lower serum sodium.

Severe hyperlipidemia causes an artifact that falsely suggests hyponatremia. In severe hyperlipidemia, as much as 20% of the plasma volume may be displaced by lipid. Sodium is dissolved only in the aqueous component of the plasma. The auto analyzers now used in hospital chemistry departments draw up a fixed volume of plasma or serum and determine the concentration of its constituents. A normal sodium concentration might then be lowered by 20%, suggesting water excess, in a patient with a marked lipid disorder. Usually, the laboratory will comment on this problem, and an osmolarity can be obtained to assess accurately the water status.

Water Depletion

Water depletion (Fig. 9–1) is recognized as an **increase in plasma sodium concentration (osmolarity)** and implies a decrease in cell water.

Causes. This disorder is relatively rare despite the large array of possible causes of water depletion (Table 9–1). **It usually develops in patients who are unable to respond to thirst because of impaired CNS function.** Normally, thirst is a powerful regulatory stimulus that effectively prevents the development of water depletion.

Clinical Findings. Symptoms, if present, reflect varying levels of **central nervous system dysfunction.** Physical signs usually are absent. In the more severe cases, the skin may become doughy and the patient irritable and depressed. **The hematocrit does not increase in water depletion because there is a proportional loss of fluid from red cells and plasma. The only criterion needed for the diagnosis of water depletion is an elevated sodium concentration (or osmolarity).**

Treatment. **Correction of water depletion includes plans for ongoing losses plus additional water for correction.** It is rarely wise to try for total correction the first

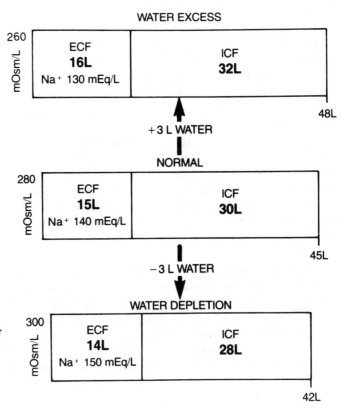

Figure 9–1. Changes that occur in ECF osmolarity, plasma sodium, and fluid compartments during water excess (**top**) and depletion (**bottom**) in a 75 kg subject.

TABLE 9–1. CAUSES OF WATER DEPLETION

I. Primary water depletion (normal renal function)
  A. Inadequate intake
    1. Coma, general anesthesia
    2. Mental obtundation
  B. Excessive losses
    1. Skin: sweating, burns
    2. Gastrointestinal: vomiting, diarrhea, bowel drainage or fistula
  C. Reset of osmoregulatory center (rare)
    1. Idiopathic
    2. Brain lesion: hydrocephalus, tumor, encephalitis
II. Functional renal impairment
  A. Concentrating defect
    1. Central diabetes insipidus (posterior pituitary defect)
    2. Nephrogenic diabetes insipidus
    3. Hypokalemic nephropathy
    4. Hypercalcemic nephropathy
  B. Osmotic diuresis
    1. Glucose
    2. Mannitol
    3. Urea

day unless deficits are small. In severe depletion in adults, an extra 1 or 2.0 L, at most, of electrolyte-free water is given daily. Infants usually are given 10 to 20 ml/kg daily. Too rapid correction of water depletion may cause convulsions because of cerebral edema.

Water Excess

Water excess is defined as a decrease in body osmolarity and implies an increase in cell water (Fig. 9–1). It is diagnosed by the finding of hyponatremia (or low osmolarity). **This is one of the most common fluid problems in hospitalized patients.**

Causes. Water excess has one basic cause, **inability of the kidney to excrete dilute urine.** In order for the kidney to excrete excess water, ADH must be suppressed. **Seriously ill or stressed individuals are unable to completely suppress ADH** secretion even in the presence of water excess.

    Hypovolemia and other low cardiac output or hypotensive states (e.g., congestive heart failure, liver failure) **are associated with increased ADH levels.** In the presence of hypotension or if plasma volume is sensed to be low, various stretch receptors (atrial, carotid sinus) signal the hypothalamus to release ADH. This volume-mediated ADH release will override osmolarity input to the hypothalamus, and progressive water retention will take place.

    In the patient with hypovolemia or low cardiac output, therefore, it only requires the administration of fluids to lead to water excess. Since many hospitalized patients are given large volumes of fluid to administer drugs and nutrients, it is not surprising that water excess is so common.

Finally, ADH may be released inappropriately (inappropriate antidiuretic hormone syndrome or IADHS) in the absence of either osmotic or volume stimuli. Sometimes pain or various drugs may stimulate pituitary release of ADH. Acute or chronic brain injury may also result in ADH release. Rarely, pituitary ADH production will occur without any known precipitating factors. In addition to pituitary sources certain tumors, particularly bronchogenic carcinoma, can synthesize ADH. Clinically IADHS is distinguished from other more common causes of ADH excess by the lack of signs of saline depletion (hypovolemia) or saline excess (edema). Urine sodium is normal in this setting as well, in contrast to the low urine sodium seen with low cardiac output or hypovolemia.

Clinical Findings. Signs and symptoms of hyponatremia often are absent, but when present, they are those of **diffuse cerebral dysfunction.** Beginning with mental confusion, these symptoms progress in severity to muscle twitching, vomiting, delirium, and finally convulsion, coma, and death. The severity of symptoms depends more on the rate of lowering of osmolarity than on the absolute level—the faster osmolarity drops (i.e., water accumulates), the more severe the symptoms.

Treatment. Therapy consists of **treating the primary cause** (e.g., hypovolemia, heart failure) whenever possible **plus restricting solute-free water intake.** This is adequate in the majority of cases. In the patient with severe hyponatremia and neurologic symptoms (obtundation, seizures), however, more rapid correction is indicated. This can be accomplished by the infusion of furosemide plus hypertonic or isotonic saline. Furosemide plus **judicious** replacement of urinary fluid losses with saline is best for emergency treatment of hypervolemic and normovolemic hyponatremia.

The extent to which body osmolarity should be raised by treatment is not clear. Usually, correcting plasma sodium to a level above 130 mEq/L is reasonable. However, some severely ill patients, when water is restricted, will develop thirst and oliguria while remaining hyponatremic. A few of these patients appear to actively regulate water balance to maintain hyposmolarity. In such patients, it is not clear which is worse, hyponatremia or thirst and oliguria. Usually, plasma creatinine and urea are normal, and there is little evidence that oliguria is harmful. The thirst can cause great discomfort. The hyponatremia usually is asymptomatic in these individuals.

SALINE DISORDERS

Physiology
The ECV is determined by the amount of sodium present in the body. Therefore, it is reasonable to describe disorders of sodium balance in terms of the size of the extracellular space. **When the patient loses sodium (usually through vomiting and diarrhea), there is contraction of the ECV.** This disorder is called **saline depletion.**

Similarly, **saline excess is present when the ECV is increased because of retention of sodium, as occurs in heart failure. The serum sodium concentration reflects water status, not saline status.** If the serum sodium is low, water is in excess. The ECV (saline) status may be high, normal, or low. Similarly, **a high serum sodium reflects water depletion.** The saline status may be high, normal, or low with water depletion as well.

Saline Depletion

Saline depletion occurs in any patient with a decrease in extracellular volume. The effect on body fluid is seen in Figure 9–2. Because **no changes in serum sodium concentration (osmolarity) have occurred, the ICV is unchanged but the ECV is smaller.** Proportionate decreases in the plasma volume also occur, since it is part of the ECV. Since red cell volume does not change, the hematocrit will increase.

Causes. The principal causes of saline loss in patients with volume depletion can be grouped into renal and nonrenal causes, as shown in Table 9–2. However, saline loss through the gastrointestinal tract is by far the most common cause of saline depletion in patients who require parenteral fluids.

The single most important criterion in the diagnosis of depletion is a **history of loss of sodium-containing fluid.** The history has both a positive and a negative value in diagnosis. On the positive side, one should suspect saline depletion in any patient who gives a history of vomiting, diarrhea, or excessive sweating or has renal salt-wasting. On the negative side, the absence of a history of loss of sodium-containing fluid makes the diagnosis of ECV depletion tenuous. These principles are based on the fact that **when the sodium intake decreases, the**

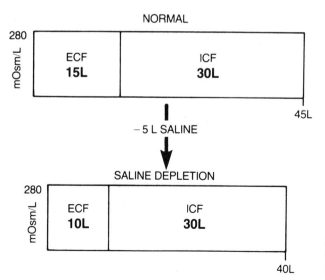

Figure 9–2. Body fluid changes following isosmolar fluid (saline) losses.

TABLE 9–2. CAUSES OF SALINE DEPLETION

I. Nonrenal losses
  A. Gastrointestinal: vomiting, diarrhea, bowel drainage, or fistula
  B. Skin: sweating, burns
  C. Iatrogenic: paracentesis, thoracentesis
II. Renal losses
  A. No intrinsic renal disease
    1. Osmotic diuresis (glucose, urea)
    2. Diuretic drugs
    3. Primary adrenal insufficiency
  B. Intrinsic renal disease
    1. Acute renal failure, diuretic phase
    2. Chronic renal failure with a sodium wasting defect (occurs in about 5% of cases).

normal kidney can conserve sodium so well that clinically detectable saline depletion does not develop. Hence, unless that patient actually loses sodium-containing fluids, he or she will not become saline depleted.

Clinical Findings. **Clinical findings in ECV depletion are primarily those of an inadequate blood volume resulting from fluid losses.** Initial symptoms of anorexia, nausea, weakness, and giddiness may be followed by orthostatic syncope and, finally, circulatory collapse.

Postural Hypotension. **Postural changes in blood pressure and heart rate are the most sensitive signs of inadequate blood volume.** When trying to elicit these diagnostic signs, it is important to measure the blood pressure and pulse first with the patient supine and then after sitting on the edge of the bed with legs dangling or standing. **Merely sitting up in bed is an insufficient postural change to elicit clinical signs of ECV depletion.** Normally, when a patient changes from the lying to the sitting or standing position, the systolic pressure changes very little, and the diastolic pressure rises about 5 to 10 mm Hg. A slight fall in systolic pressure alone does not indicate an inadequate blood volume.

    Significant postural hypotension also occurs in the presence of severe peripheral autonomic nervous system disease and in some cardiac patients with a fixed cardiac output.

Neck Veins. **The jugular venous pressure is another useful clinical indicator of the blood volume (and therefore of the ECV).** When a patient lies absolutely flat on his or her back, the neck veins should be full nearly to the angle of the jaw. If the bed must be raised before a level can be seen, the pressure is increased, and blood volume overload should be suspected. The finding of decreased filling or **flat neck veins** that fill only when compressed at the clavicle **strongly suggests an inadequate blood volume.**

Urine Volume. **Hourly urine output is also an indication of the adequacy of blood volume.** However, its value is limited because oliguria may be caused by a wide variety of problems. The circumstances in which urine volume is most helpful are the following.

1. If during volume replacement there is an increase in hourly urine volume from oliguric levels of 0 to 10 mL/hour up to 50 mL/hour or more, an adequate blood volume has been restored.
2. In patients who are losing blood volume rapidly (gastrointestinal bleeding or severe burns), a drop in the hourly urine volume usually indicates that volume replacement is not keeping up with losses.

Other Conditions. Several other clinical states may present findings suggestive of ECV depletion. In Table 9–3, the major entities that may confuse us are presented. Helpful distinguishing features are as follows.

1. **Acute blood loss** shows all the dynamic features of ECV depletion. Usually, some **evidence of bleeding** will be present to clarify the situation. Occasionally, an abdominal catastrophe (vessel rupture or large gastrointestinal bleeding episode) will be difficult to recognize.
2. **Septic shock** presents many objective features that resemble ECV depletion. Curiously, **fever may not be present at the outset** when shock is most severe (on the contrary, many patients are hypothermic). Two features frequently are helpful. Unlike individuals with other causes of shock, these patients are **vasodilated.** Their extremities are warm, and **urine output is normal or even increased.**
3. **Myocardial infarction** often has all the features of ECV depletion, except that these patients usually have **elevated neck veins.** Edema may be present as well.
4. **Hypoalbuminemia** also can be very confusing. Severe hypoalbuminemia leads to low intravascular volume with the features of ECV depletion. **Edema,** however, is also present and should strongly suggest (with volume depletion) that hypoalbuminemia is present.

Treatment. Therapy consists of giving an **isotonic sodium solution. The more certain the evidence that volume depletion is present, the more vigorous replacement therapy should be.** Although it is true that acute pulmonary edema may result from overly rapid administration of saline, it is equally true that unnecessary prolongation of hypovolemia by too slow replacement of the saline deficit can

TABLE 9–3. COMMON CLINICAL CONDITIONS THAT SIMULATE ECV DEPLETION

Condition	Blood Pressure	Orthostatic BP Change	Neck Veins	Urine Output	Edema
Acute blood loss	Low	Present	Low	Low	Absent
Septic shock	Low	Present	Low	High	Absent
Myocardial infarct	Low	Present	High	Low	Variable
Hypoalbuminemia	Variable	Variable	Variable	Variable	Present

have disastrous consequences, especially if the patient is stressed by surgery or

In the presence of volume depletion, intravenous administration of saline can proceed as rapidly as 1 L/hour or, in severe cases, even faster, provided that the physician monitors the patient frequently. As soon as the signs of severe hypovolemia begin to disappear, the rate of saline replacement is slowed.

Only a rough estimate of the severity of saline depletion is necessary. **Severe depletion usually is associated with low blood pressure and flat neck veins even when the patient is supine. Often the blood pressure is unobtainable when the patient sits up. These findings represent an ECV depletion of 50% or greater.**

Patients with moderate depletion, documented by orthostatic blood pressure changes and visible but low neck veins, have an ECV depletion in the neighborhood of 25%. Since the ECV is normally about 20% of the body weight, such information provides a guide to the amount of correction needed.

Saline Excess

Causes. **Heart failure, liver disease, renal failure, and nephrotic syndrome are common causes of saline excess. However, in the hospitalized patient receiving intravenous fluid therapy, the most common cause is iatrogenic.** Seriously ill patients often cannot excrete normal saline loads (200 to 300 mEq/day of sodium is contained in a normal diet). Hence, it is easy to overload such patients, and this often happens in hospital practice.

Fortunately, moderate saline excess, as represented by minimal sacral edema in the prone patient, seldom causes serious problems. **It usually requires a 3 to 6 L increase in the ECV to produce detectable sacral edema in a bedridden patient.** Lower leg edema is a less reliable guide to the presence of saline excess, since local venous obstruction and postural changes can cause local edema without an increase in the overall ECV. The changes that occur with saline excess in the body fluid compartments are noted in Figure 9–3.

Clinical Findings. **Edema is the principal physical finding in saline excess.** If edema is present and is not due to local factors (e.g., varicose veins), saline excess exists. Elevated neck veins and increased blood pressure also may occur, but these findings are not necessary for the diagnosis.

The hematocrit often is normal because saline excess develops rather slowly, and compensatory factors maintain the hematocrit. **The urine sodium or chloride usually is low because the same factors that cause edema also cause renal retention of sodium and chloride.** Were it not for renal retention of sodium, the disorder would be corrected quickly. **As in saline depletion, the serum sodium concentration is normal.**

Treatment. There are three considerations in the therapy of saline excess.

1. Treatment of the underlying cause (e.g., heart failure, hypoproteinemia)
2. Sodium restriction is necessary
3. Diuretics often are indicated

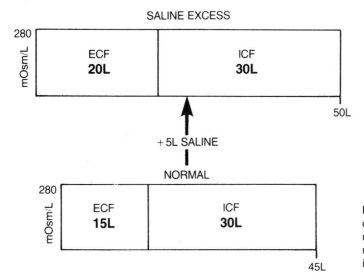

Figure 9–3. Expansion of ECF due to isosmolar saline retention. This usually is manifested by edema or increased transcellular fluid.

The "Third Space" Problem. Some patients have clinical signs of **hypovolemia** despite findings of an **excessive sequestration of saline** in some area of the body. **This area of fluid accumulation is referred to as a third space to distinguish it from the ICV and ECV.** Actually, third space fluid is a part of the ECV.

The third space may be a segment of the normal ECV, for example, the edema that occurs in an extremity after thrombophlebitis, surgical removal of lymph nodes, or a thermal burn. It also may be due to loculation of transcellular fluid in the gut secondary to obstruction or excessive peritoneal or pleural fluid.

Initially, accumulation of fluid in this third space occurs at the expense of the plasma volume. Hence, many patients **show signs of hypovolemia** (flat neck veins, postural hypotension, low urine sodium concentration) **despite weight gain and an obvious collection of excess body fluid.**

The normal physiologic response to a loss of fluid from the plasma volume into the third space is a decrease in renal sodium excretion as an attempt to restore the effective ECV to normal. **It is important that the weight gain caused by sodium and water loculation not be mistaken for an increase in effective ECV and treated with sodium restriction or diuretics because the result will be hypovolemia and hypotension, with little decrease in the third space.**

PRACTICAL MANAGEMENT OF FLUID AND ELECTROLYTE DISORDERS

There are three steps to the practical approach to management: (1) determine the basic allowance, (2) establish the diagnosis, and (3) determine the treatment.

Determine the Basic Allowance

The basic allowance is that amount of fluid and electrolytes necessary to maintain the status quo. To estimate the basic allowance one must consider the routes of loss and replace these. Typical basic allowances for an adult are shown in Table 9–4. These are the anticipated losses that will be replaced.

Urinary Loss of Fluid and Electrolytes

1. **In most clinical situations, the urine basic allowance** will be constant as shown **(1500 ml)** except in two settings.
2. With urine volume less than 500 mL/24 hours, the actual volume of urine lost is used in the basic allowance, with proportional reductions in electrolytes.
3. With urine volumes in excess of 3000 mL/24 hours, the actual volume of urine lost should be used in planning treatment for the next 24 hours. In this situation, if possible, urine electrolytes should be measured as well and the actual amount that is lost given as replacement. If the electrolytes have not been measured, the **electrolyte replacement should be proportionately increased.**

Sensible and Insensible (S & I) Losses. This loss is usually estimated at 1000 mL/24 hours. This fluid is lost by **evaporation through the skin and lungs.** S & I loss is altered in two settings: (1) when a patient is on a ventilator, humidified air generally is used, and little or no water is lost with breathing. Therefore, the sensible and insensible losses will be decreased by about 50%, and only 500 mL should be provided for this loss. If the patient has a high fever or, for some reason, is in a hot environment, these losses will be higher. **Typically, S & I loss should be increased by 50% for fever > 39°C (102°F) or environmental temperature > 30°C (80°F).**

Gastrointestinal Losses. These usually are constant. Therefore, when such losses occur, the traditional practice is to give in the next 24 hours the volume lost in the last 24 hours. Electrolyte losses with gastrointestinal fluids usually are replaced according to Table 9–5, but sometimes they are measured, and the measured losses are replaced. Gastric losses are assumed to have equal sodium and chloride

TABLE 9–4. AVERAGE DAILY BASIC ALLOWANCES

Output	Water mL	Sodium mEq	Chloride mEq	Potassium mEq
Urine	1500	50	90	40
Sensible and insensible	1000	0	0	0
Gastrointestinal	Previous volume + trend	Equal or half Cl	100 mEq/L or measured	10 mEq/L

TABLE 9-5. TYPICAL COMPOSITION OF GASTROINTESTINAL FLUIDS IN ADULT

Type	Volume^a	Na$^+$	K^{+b}	Cl^{-b}	HCO$_3^-$	pH^{+b}
Gastric	Measured	40–100	10	100	0	1–6
Bile	0.5–1.0	145	5	110	40	7–8
Pancreatic	1.0–2.0	140	10	50	100	7–8
Diarrheal	Measured	80–120	10	80–120	0–20	4–8

^{a}L/day
^{b}mEq/L

concentrations if the pH is relatively high (>4). With lower pHs, sodium may be assumed to be half the standard chloride loss.

Establish the Diagnosis

Principles. **Saline status must be established as normal, increased, or decreased.** Consideration must be given to the total extracellular volume, intravascular volume, and potential third space problems.

1. Edema means saline excess
2. Saline is lost from the ECV
3. Hypotension, orthostatic hypotension, or low neck veins suggest intravascular volume deficit
4. Edema accompanied by intravascular volume deficit suggests hypoalbuminemia

Water status must be established as normal, increased, or decreased.

1. Serum sodium concentration (corrected for glucose if necessary) reflects osmolarity
   a. Low sodium means water excess
   b. High sodium means water depletion
2. Water is lost from both ICV and ECV—two thirds from ICV, one third from ECV
3. Water abnormalities appear clinically as brain dysfunction

Correct the Abnormalities

Principles. **For each disorder, specific therapy must be applied.** Some estimate of the severity of the disorder must be made to calculate corrections. In general, severe abnormalities will require larger corrections.

Body Weight and Serum Sodium as a Guide to ICV and ECV Status. **Changes in body weight over a short period of time measure changes in total body water.** Hence, to use body weight as a guide to saline need, a way of calculating changes in ECV from the observed change in body weight must be formulated. The following equation indicates the components of body weight change.

$$\text{Weight} = \text{ECV} + \text{ICV} + \text{nonfluid mass}$$

Since ECV usually is the desired measurement, a method of estimating ICV and nonfluid mass is needed. To estimate ICV, two assumptions are necessary.

1. The ICV can be estimated as about 40% of the body weight
2. Changes in the ICV are proportional to changes in plasma sodium concentration (plasma osmolality)

$$\Delta \text{ICV} = \text{normal ICV} \times \text{percent change in plasma sodium concentration}$$
$$= (0.4 \times \text{body weight}) \times \frac{\text{initial} - \text{final } [Na^+]_p}{\text{initial } [Na^+]_p}$$

where $[Na^+]_p$ = sodium concentration in plasma.

Example

Parameter	Initial	Final
Weight, kg	70	75
$[Na^+]_p$, mEq/L	140	140

$$\Delta \text{Weight} = \Delta \text{ECV} + \Delta \text{ICV}$$
$$+5 = \Delta \text{ECV} + (0.4 \times 70) \times \frac{140 - 140}{140}$$

$$+5 = \Delta \text{ECV} + 0$$
$$\Delta \text{ECV} = +5 \text{ L}$$

In this example, the lack of variation in the plasma sodium concentration indicated that no change occurred in the ICV. Therefore, the entire weight change was due to an increase (5 L) in the ECV. In acute situations, nonfluid mass change is negligible, so this was not included here.

Example

Parameter	Initial	Final
Weight, kg	60	62.5
$[Na^+]_p$, mEq/L	135	125

$$\Delta \text{Weight} = \Delta \text{ECV} + \Delta \text{ICV}$$
$$+2.5 = \Delta \text{ECV} + (0.4 \times 60) \times \frac{135 - 125}{135}$$

$$+2.5 = \Delta \text{ECV} + 1.8$$
$$\Delta \text{ECV} = +0.7 \text{ L}$$

In this instance, the weight gain (2.5 kg) was due to an increase in both ICV (1.8 L) and ECV (0.7 L) from water excess, which resulted in a fall in body osmolarity.

Nonfluid Mass. In patients receiving inadequate calories, a common situation in ill, hospitalized patients, an estimation of the weight loss due to decrease in nonfluid mass (fat and nonfat solids) is made by assuming a **0.3 kg/day decrease**. In catabolic patients, this loss may be as great as 0.6 kg/day.

Example. A patient is on intravenous fluids for 4 days.

Parameter	Initial	Final
Weight, kg	70	70
$[Na^+]_p$, mEq/L	135	135

$$\Delta \text{ Weight} = \Delta \text{ ECV} + \Delta \text{ ICV} + \Delta \text{ nonfluid mass}$$
$$0 = \Delta \text{ ECV} + 0 + (-0.3 \text{ kg/day} \times 4 \text{ days})$$
$$\Delta \text{ ECV} = +1.2 \text{ L}$$

The patient should have lost weight during the 4 days on parenteral fluids. The stable body weight without change in the plasma sodium concentration means the ECV has increased.

Treatment Guidelines

1. Include **basic allowance** in all cases
2. **Correct intravascular volume deficit first, quickly**
3. **Correct water abnormalities slowly.** Except with CNS dysfunction, a brief rapid correction (e.g., 10 mEq Na^+ change in 10 hours) should be followed by a slow correction.
4. Treat a **third space as saline loss**
5. **When water excess and saline depletion are combined, treating the saline depletion will allow the body to correct the water excess.**

STUDY CASES

Case 1

This is an example of how the steps in formulating a plan to therapy are applied.

History. A 67-year-old woman had an elective cholecystectomy. On the fourth post-operative day, she developed nausea, vomiting, and ileus, with minimal abdominal distention.

Physical Examination. Weight 48 kg (2 kg less than on admission), temperature 36.8°C, respiration 15, pulse 82, blood pressure 150/85 lying and 145/90 sitting. Neck veins were full in supine position. Heart and lungs were unchanged from previous examinations.

Laboratory Data. Hct 40%, WBC 11,100, serum sodium 147, potassium 4.2, chloride 110, bicarbonate (CO_2)* 24 mEq/L, urea nitrogen 10, creatinine 0.8, and glucose 95

---

* Some laboratories refer to this term as a bicarbonate, others as CO_2, total CO_2 or carbon dioxide. We find these latter terms are easily confused with P_{CO_2} and therefore avoid them.

mg/dL. Urine output (24 hours) was 600 mL, and the first 6 hours of nasogastric suction produced 500 mL at a pH of 6.

Basic Allowance. The estimated (urine, S & I) or measured gastrointestinal basic allowances are shown in the worksheet. Note first of all that the basic allowance for urine water is 1500 mL rather than the volume of 600 mL recorded for the previous day. The reasoning here is that the oliguria represents an attempt by the kidneys to conserve water and help correct a water deficit. If a basic urine allowance of 600 mL was made, the kidneys would not have the opportunity to help in further correction of a water deficit should it continue. Similarly, the basic allowances for sodium, chloride, and potassium in the urine are not the output from the previous day, which, in the case of sodium and potassium, is unknown. Instead, the basic allowances for urinary electrolytes, following the principles previously outlined, are 50 for sodium, 40 for potassium, and 90 for chloride. S & I allowance is simply 1000 mL of water. As shown in the worksheet, no allowance is made for S & I loss of electrolyte unless sweating is anticipated, which is not the case here. Basic allowance for gastrointestinal loss is based on the output during the first few hours. In this case, the output is 500 mL in 6 hours (estimate 2000 mL in 24 hours).

Since the gastric fluid pH was 6, the sodium concentration was assumed to be 100 mEq. This is assumed also to be the concentration in the next 24 hours, giving a total of 200 mEq/L. Since the pH of the fluid is 6, the output of sodium can be expected roughly equal the output of chloride, so the total is also 200. Potassium figured at the rate of 10 mEq/L becomes 20 for the basic allowance. These allowances are now totaled as shown: 4500 mL for water, 250 mEq for sodium, 60 mEq for potassium, and 310 mEq for chloride. These totals represent the amount of fluid and electrolyte that the patient needs during the next 24 hours to maintain the status quo. At the same time, these allowances provide the kidney with optimum amounts of fluid and electrolytes to correct subclinical imbalances.

Correction of Disorders. The diagnosis of water depletion is made on the basis of a serum sodium level of 147mEq/L. Thirst, oliguria, and high urine osmolarity might also suggest the diagnosis. Therefore, a correction allowance of 1 L of water is made. The columns are then totaled, and the planned intake is determined as this total. The planned intake of chloride is equal to the sum of sodium and potassium.

BASIC ALLOWANCE

	Volume	Na+	K+	H+	Cl-	HCO3-
Urine	1500	50	40	▨	90	▨
S + I	1000	▨	▨	▨	▨	▨
GI	2000	200	20		220	
TOTAL:	4500	250	60		310	

Worksheet 9–1. Fluid balance worksheet, Case 1, answers.

DIAGNOSES:
1. ECV (Saline) NORMAL
2. Water DEPLETION
3. Acid/Base NORMAL
4. Potassium NORMAL

Corrections	Volume	Na+	K+	H+	Cl-	HCO3-
Saline +/-			▓▓▓	▓▓▓		▓▓▓
Water +/-	+1000	▓▓▓	▓▓▓	▓▓▓	▓▓▓	▓▓▓
Acid/Base +/-						
Potassium +/-	▓▓▓	▓▓▓				
SUM: Basics + Corrections	5500	250	60		310	

Worksheet 9–1. Continued.

Case 2

History. A 43-year-old housewife, previously in good health, developed an acute illness characterized by adominal cramps, nausea, vomiting, and diarrhea. About 36 hours after the onset of her symptoms, she was hospitalized on 10/1. At this time, her cramps and diarrhea had subsided, but vomiting persisted.

Physical Examination. Weight 61.5 kg (usual 63.5 kg), temperature 37° C, respiration 18, pulse 92, blood pressure 100/60 (supine). Neck veins were not visible when she was supine. Blood pressure while sitting was 70/20, with an increase in pulse rate to 105. The abdomen was distended and tympanitic and had active bowel sounds.

Laboratory Data. Hct 50% (usual 40%), WBC 10,500, serum sodium 135, potassium 3.5, chloride 98, HCO_3^- 24 mEq/L, glucose 85, urea nitrogen 35, creatinine 1.2 mg/dL, albumin 3.6 g/dL. Urine output was not recorded, but the patient had voided several times.

1. What fluid and electrolyte disorders are present? Estimate the severity of the ECV depletion.

A tube for nasogastric suction was placed, and the patient was started on intravenous fluids. Over the next 24 hours, she received 6000 mL of fluid containing 600 mEq of NaCl and 60 mEq of KCl. Her urine output was 2200 mL, and her nasogastric suction produced 1500 mL. On 10/2, the laboratory values were Hct 39%, serum sodium 134, potassium 3.5, chloride 98, HCO_3^- 25 mEq/L, glucose 95, urea nitrogen 20, creatinine 1.0 mg/dL. Blood pressure was 110/70 without postural fall, and neck veins were now visible. Weight was 63 kg. The abdomen was less distended.

2. What is the fluid and electrolyte status at present?
3. Estimate the change in her ECF volume and blood volume from 10/1 to 10/2.
4. Plan treatment for the next 24 hours, using the worksheet on the next page.

BASIC ALLOWANCE						
	Volume	Na+	K+	H+	Cl-	HCO3-
Urine				▨		▨
S + I		▨	▨	▨	▨	▨
GI						
TOTAL:						

DIAGNOSES:
1. ECV (Saline)
2. Water
3. Acid/Base
4. Potassium

Corrections	Volume	Na+	K+	H+	Cl-	HCO3-
Saline +/-			▨	▨		▨
Water +/-		▨	▨	▨	▨	▨
Acid/Base +/-						
Potassium +/-	▨	▨				
SUM: Basics + Corrections						

Case 3

History. A mildly demented 72-year-old woman was admitted from a nursing home because of increasing lethargy, anorexia, and failure to thrive.

Physical Examination. Her weight was 52 kg (usually about 55 kg), temperature 37.5°C, pulse 90 and irregular, respiration 16, blood pressure 180/90 lying and 170/95 sitting. She appeared cachectic and somnolent. Skin turgor was poor, but her tongue was normal. Neck veins were full when supine. Chest, heart, abdomen, and neurologic examinations were normal.

Laboratory Data. Hct 35%, WBC 8500, serum sodium 155, potassium 4.5, chloride 116, HCO$_3^-$ 28 mEq/L, glucose 82, urea nitrogen 16, and creatinine 1.0 mg/dL. Urinalysis: specific gravity 1.020, protein, glucose, blood negative, ketones positive, sediment unremarkable.

5. What fluid and electrolyte problems are present?
6. Quantify any imbalances noted.
7. Describe the pathogenesis of the fluid and electrolyte problems found in this patient.
8. Plan treatment using the worksheet on the next page.

BASIC ALLOWANCE

	Volume	Na+	K+	H+	Cl-	HCO3-
Urine				▩		▩
S + I		▩	▩	▩	▩	
GI						
TOTAL:						

DIAGNOSES:
1. ECV (Saline)
2. Water
3. Acid/Base
4. Potassium

Corrections	Volume	Na+	K+	H+	Cl-	HCO3-
Saline +/-			▩			▩
Water +/-		▩	▩	▩	▩	▩
Acid/Base +/-						
Potassium +/-	▩	▩				
SUM: Basics + Corrections						

Case 4

History. A 65-year-old man was admitted for shortness of breath. He had recently stopped taking his usual medication (digoxin and hydrochlorothiazide). He says he may have gained weight, but he has no scale at home.

Physical Examination. His weight was 78 kg, temperature 37.5°C, blood pressure 130/78 without postural changes, normal vital signs. He had bibasilar rales, and cardiac examination revelealed an S3 gallop. He had mild pitting edema of the ankles. The remainder of the examination was unremarkable.

Laboratory Data. Chest x-ray showed cardiomegaly and some pulmonary edema. Hct 40%, sodium 130, potassium 3.9, chloride 95, HCO_3^- 25, urea nitrogen 30, creatinine 1.0, and glucose 100. He had voided twice on the day of admission.

   9. What fluid and electrolyte disorders are present?
   10. Plan therapy for the next 24 hours, using the worksheet on the next page.

BASIC ALLOWANCE						
	Volume	Na+	K+	H+	Cl-	HCO3-
Urine				▓▓▓▓		▓▓▓▓
S + I		▓▓▓▓▓▓▓▓▓▓▓▓▓▓▓▓▓▓▓▓▓▓				
GI						
TOTAL:						

DIAGNOSES:
1. ECV (Saline)
2. Water
3. Acid/Base
4. Potassium

Corrections	Volume	Na+	K+	H+	Cl-	HCO3-
Saline +/-			▓▓▓▓▓▓▓▓▓▓			▓▓▓▓
Water +/-		▓▓▓▓▓▓▓▓▓▓▓▓▓▓▓▓▓▓▓▓▓▓▓▓				
Acid/Base +/-						
Potassium +/-	▓▓▓▓▓▓▓▓▓▓▓▓					
SUM: Basics + Corrections						

ANSWERS TO STUDY CASES

Case 2

1. What fluid and electrolyte disorders are present? Estimate the severity of the ECV depletion.

ECF. The low blood pressure with postural hypotension, flat neck veins, and elevated hematocrit are consistent with an **acute** reduction of the blood volume. The weight loss and history suggest salt and water loss from the gastrointestinal tract. The distended, tympanitic abdomen suggests a third space problem with extra fluid in the bowel.

Water. The serum sodium and glucose concentrations are normal. Therefore, no osmolar disturbance is present.

Acid-base. The serum HCO_3^- and anion gap are normal. This suggests that no significant acid-base disorder is present.

Potassium. The serum potassium is mildly low, but in the absence of an arterial pH, it is difficult to quantitate the degree of possible deficit. This history of vomiting and diarrhea suggests losses from the gastrointestinal tract (potassium problems are considered in Chapter 10).

2. What is the fluid and electrolyte status at present?

ECF. The large amount of saline administered was helpful in correcting the ECF depletion.

Water. Little change occurred.

Acid-base. No significant change occurred.

Potassium. There was no significant improvement despite administration of 60 mEq.

3. Estimate the change in her ECF volume and blood volume from 10/1 to 10/2.

$$\Delta \text{ Body weight } = \Delta \text{ ECF } + \Delta \text{ ICF}$$
$$+1.5L = \Delta \text{ ECF } + \frac{(135 - 134)}{135} \times (0.4 \times 61.5)$$
$$+1.3L = \Delta \text{ ECF}$$
$$\Delta \text{ Blood volume } = \Delta \text{ Hct}$$
$$= \frac{50 - 39}{50}$$

= 0.22, or 22% decrease in hematocrit caused by reciprocal increase in blood volume.

4. Plan a treatment for the next 24 hours.

See fluid balance worksheet 9–2. Note that although the patient put out 2200 mL of urine, only 1500 mL were replaced. This approach allows the body's physiology to participate in the corrections. If urine output were matched each day, one could wind up like the cat chasing its tail. Some potassium correction has been made (see chapter 10).

BASIC ALLOWANCE

	Volume	Na+	K+	H+	Cl-	HCO3-
Urine	1500	50	40		90	
S + I	1000					
GI	1500	150	15		165	
TOTAL:	4000	200	55		255	

140 PRACTICAL FLUIDS AND ELECTROLYTES

DIAGNOSES:
1. ECV (Saline) NORMAL
2. Water NORMAL
3. Acid/Base NORMAL
4. Potassium SLIGHT DEPLETION

Corrections	Volume	Na+	K+	H+	Cl-	HCO3-
Saline +/-						
Water +/-						
Acid/Base +/-						
Potassium +/-			(50)		(50)	
SUM: Basics + Corrections	4000	200	105		305	

Worksheet 9–2. Fluid balance worksheet, Case 2, answers.

Case 3

5. What fluid and electrolyte problems are present?

ECF (Saline). Except for poor skin turgor, which is probably caused by aging and loss of elastic tissue, there are no findings of significant depletion.

Water. The serum sodium concentration is elevated and indicates depletion with intracellular contraction.

Acid-base. No changes noted.

Potassium. No changes noted.

6. Quantify any imbalances noted.

$$\Delta \text{ Water} = \frac{\text{Present serum sodium} - \text{initial serum sodium}}{\text{Initial serum sodium}} \times \text{TBW}$$

$$\frac{155 - 140}{140} \times (0.6 \times 55) = 3.5 \text{ L deficit}$$

This formula is similar to the one previously shown but uses total body water (60% of weight, both ECV and ICV). When saline status appears reasonable, this is a useful shortcut.

7. Describe the pathogenesis of the fluid and electrolyte problems.

The most likely cause (Table 9–4) would be inadequate intake. The urine specific gravity of 1.020 and lack of glucosuria eliminate a lack of ADH or nephrogenic causes. Many old people in nursing facilities are unable to communicate their feelings of thirst and also may not physically be able to obtain water on their own.

BASIC ALLOWANCE

	Volume	Na+	K+	H+	Cl-	HCO3-
Urine	1500	50	40	▨	90	▨
S + I	1000	▨	▨	▨	▨	▨
GI						
TOTAL:	2500	50	40		90	

DIAGNOSES:
1. ECV (Saline) NORMAL
2. Water DEFICIT
3. Acid/Base NORMAL
4. Potassium NORMAL

Corrections	Volume	Na+	K+	H+	Cl-	HCO3-
Saline +/-			▨	▨		▨
Water +/-	+1500	▨	▨	▨	▨	▨
Acid/Base +/-						
Potassium +/-	▨	▨				
SUM: Basics + Corrections	4000	50	40		90	

Worksheet 9–3. Fluid balance worksheet, Case 3, answers.

8. Plan treatment using the worksheet.

There is no reason to change the daily basic allowances for this patient. An attempt should be made to slowly correct her water deficit. As noted previously, no attempt is made to give a total correction on the first day. An extra 1 or 2 L, at most, of electrolyte-free water daily can be given until correction is completed. This rule prevents a too rapid fall in serum sodium, which could cause headache and, in extreme cases, convulsions from brain swelling (Worksheet 9–3).

Case 4

9. What fluid and electrolyte disorders are present?

ECF. The patient's history suggests the possibility of saline retention. Examination (rales, gallop, edema) seems to confirm this. Without knowing his baseline weight, we cannot be sure of the amount, but at his size, it takes at least 3L of saline excess to become clinically apparent.

Water. The low sodium means water has been retained in excess of the sodium.

Low cardiac output leads to water retention by stimulating ADH through volume receptors. The exact amount cannot be estimated accurately without knowing his baseline serum sodium, and weight, but assuming a value of 140mEq/L as normal, his water excess amounts to at least 3L.

10. Plan a therapy for the next 24 hours.

Therapy would not require intravenous fluids, but the same principles can be used with oral fluids. In this patient, the reinstitution of diuretics should be combined with dietary sodium restriction. The mild water excess does not need treatment but should be monitored. Because the diuretics may eliminate more sodium than he takes in, a negative sodium balance could be achieved in such a situation. (Worksheet 9–4).

BASIC ALLOWANCE

	Volume	Na+	K+	H+	Cl-	HCO3-
Urine	1500	50	40	/////	90	/////
S + I	1000	/////	/////	/////	/////	/////
GI						
TOTAL:	2500	50	40		90	

DIAGNOSES:
1. ECV (Saline) EXCESS
2. Water EXCESS (slight)
3. Acid/Base NORMAL
4. Potassium NORMAL

Corrections	Volume	Na+	K+	H+	Cl-	HCO3-
Saline +/-	-300	50	/////		50	/////
Water +/-		/////	/////	/////	/////	/////
Acid/Base +/-						
Potassium +/-	/////	/////				
SUM: Basics + Corrections	2200	0	40		40	

Worksheet 9–4. Fluid balance worksheet, Case 4, answers.

Potassium

INTRODUCTION

Potassium is the major intracellular cation. Its movement between ECF and ICF is influenced by pH and insulin. With normal pH and glucose-insulin metabolism, the serum potassium level reflects total body potassium stores. Whereas the major extracellular cation, sodium, determines the extracellular volume, variations in potassium do not influence intracellular volume. Alterations in potassium cause two major problems:

1. By its influence on cell depolarization, potassium abnormalities result in disturbances in striated muscle and nerves. Most importantly, **cardiac arrhythmias and cardiac arrest** occur in patients with potassium disorders.
2. Although the exact mechanisms are unclear, changes in potassium content affect pH. **Potassium depletion can cause alkalosis, whereas potassium excess may contribute to acidosis.**

STUDY OBJECTIVES

To understand the

1. Causes
2. Consequences
3. Diagnosis
4. Management

of the following conditions

1. Potassium depletion
2. Potassium excess

PHYSIOLOGY

Quantitation of Potassium Disorders

The plasma potassium concentration, properly interpreted, is an accurate guide to the potassium needs of the patient. **A high serum potassium usually reflects potassium excess, whereas a low serum potassium implies potassium depletion.**

Interpretation of Plasma Potassium Concentration. Using the plasma potassium level to quantitate potassium need is fairly simple, provided the following points are kept in mind.

1. The magnitude of the disorder must be related to the size of the patient, or more accurately, to the normal total body potassium
2. The normal relationship between plasma potassium level and its intracellular concentration is semilogarithmic
3. Changes in acid-base balance can affect the plasma potassium level independent of need
4. About 98% of the total body potassium is intracellular

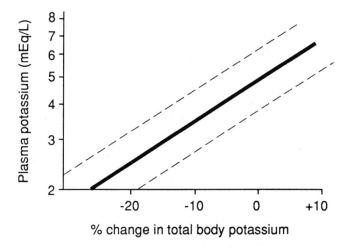

Figure 10–1. The exponential relationship of plasma potassium concentration to changes in body potassium content and capacity.

There is a **rough quantitative relationship between** plasma potassium **and potassium depletion or excess.** The plasma potassium concentration on a logarithmic scale is proportional to the total body potassium (Figure 10–1). Thus, the plasma potassium concentration defines a potassium disorder as the percent deviation from normal. If the total body potassium were known, the milliequivalents of potassium depletion or excess could be calculated. **A reasonable estimation of total potassium can be made from a simple estimation of the degree of muscle mass based on body weight (Table 10–1).**

Example: A male patient weighs 70 kg. He has lost 4 kg during his present illness and appears to be slightly malnourished. His plasma potassium is 2.8 mEq/L. The estimated total body potassium is 70 kg × 30 mEq/kg, or 2100 mEq (from Table 10–1). Figure 10–1 shows that at this plasma level, the depletion is about 17%, or about 350 mEq (0.17 × 2100 = 357). If about 350 mEq of potassium is given, the serum potassium should normalize.

Only a very rough estimation of potassium deficit is needed, since serial measurments of the plasma potassium level are used to guide and monitor replacement therapy.

Effect of Acid-Base Imbalance on Plasma Potassium. Changes in extracellular pH affect the internal equilibrium between the plasma potassium concentration and the intracellular potassium concentration. **Acidosis increases the plasma potassium level, and alkalosis decreases the plasma potassium level.** A possible

TABLE 10–1. ESTIMATION OF TOTAL BODY POTASSIUM

	Males mEq/kg	Females mEq/kg
Normal	45	35
Moderate wasting	30	25
Very marked wasting	20	20

explanation is that changes in intracellular hydrogen ion change the cellular potassium capacity. **The practical consequence is that the plasma potassium level accurately reflects the intracellular or total body potassium only if there is no acid-base disorder.** Corrections must be applied when an acid-base abnormality also is present. This means that **with a reduced blood pH (acidosis), a normal plasma potassium level signifies depletion and a low plasma level reflects severe depletion. When blood pH is high (alkalosis), normal intracellular potassium stores are associated with a low plasma potassium level.**

A rough assessment of the influence of acid-base disorders on the relationship between the plasma potassium and intracellular potassium is necessary if plasma potassium is to be used as a guide to potassium therapy. This relationship is indicated in Figure 10–2, which depicts the influence of blood pH on plasma potassium with no change in total potassium stores. **Each 0.1 of a unit change in blood pH results in a change of about 0.7 mEq/L in the plasma potassium.** This degree of change is typical of situations involving the addition or loss of HCl or HCO_3^- from the body. When an organic acidosis (e.g., diabetic ketoacidosis) occurs, the effect on potassium is somewhat less. In addition, with extreme changes of either acid-base or potassium balance, the relationship tends to be less precise.

Clinical Use of the Plasma Potassium Level. The significance of the plasma potassium level cannot be underestimated. **Plasma potassium usually reflects total body potassium, and an alteration in total body potassium eventually must be corrected to correct the plasma potassium.** Nonetheless, the plasma (ECV) potassium is most important in determining membrane polarity. Deviation in plasma potassium, hypokalemia (low) or hyperkalemia (high), must be avoided or corrected.

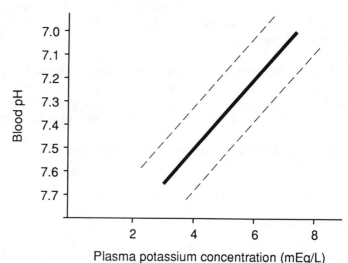

Figure 10–2. The effect of changes in blood pH on plasma potassium concentration.

Example: A 40-year-old woman enters the hospital with vomiting of 3 days duration (vomiting may lead to large hydrogen ion loss, but usually not much potassium loss). Plasma potassium is 3.0 mEq/L, and blood pH is 7.60. Reference to Figure 10–2 shows that this is about what would be expected if there were no potassium disorder. Her plasma potassium should be corrected to 4.5 mEq/L if the alkalosis is corrected to a blood pH of 7.40.

Potassium Balance

Intake

Diet. **The typical diet contains about 100 mEq of potassium daily**. Vegetarians may have considerably higher intakes, and herbiverous animals may consume 10 times this amount.

Tissues. Normally, anabolism and catabolism are in balance, and newly formed cells take up the potassium lost as senescent cells die. With marked tissue injury (e.g., a crush injury) or in catabolic states, a larger amount of potassium may enter the system from tissue destruction than is used in tissue regeneration.

Excretion

Normal. The major sites by which potassium leaves the body are the kidney, which accounts for 90% of potassium excretion, and the gut and skin (sweat), which together account for 10% of potassium excretion. **Gut and sweat losses are fixed, but the kidney can reduce its loss in states of depletion to about 5% of the average.** Thus, there is an approximate 10 mEq daily loss of potassium in the absence of any intake. As a result, potassium depletion will slowly develop in the absence of any intake.

Abnormalities. **Abnormalities of potassium balance usually result from excretory abnormalities.** Excessive losses from gut or kidney cause depletion, whereas failure of renal excretion is the usual cause of potassium overload.

POTASSIUM DEPLETION

Potassium depletion is defined as decreased total body potassium. Depletion should be suspected by **historical** circumstances that commonly lead to a negative balance, such as **poor dietary intake or excessive losses from the gut and kidneys** (Table 10–2).

Causes

Inadequate Diet (Intake). Because of normal renal and gut losses, a **prolonged** inadequate diet may result in potassium deficiency.

TABLE 10–2. PRINCIPAL CAUSES OF POTASSIUM DEPLETION

I. Deficient dietary intake
II. Excessive Losses
    A. Gastrointestinal
        1. Protracted vomiting
        2. Diarrhea
        3. Fistula
        4. Laxative abuse
    B. Renal
        1. Metabolic alkalosis
        2. Diuretics
        3. Aldosteronism
        4. Tubular dysfunction

Excessive Losses

Gastrointestinal Losses. **Vomiting** will result in modest losses that may become significant if prolonged. More important as a cause of potassium loss is the resultant **metabolic alkalosis,** which not only causes a shift of potassium into cells but also induces excessive renal losses.

Diarrhea from any cause, including malabsorption, enteritis, or laxative abuse, may lead to depletion because of the loss of large volumes of **potassium-rich (20 to 40 mEq/L) fluid.**

Fistulous tracts from almost anywhere in the gastrointestinal system will lead to potassium depletion if large volumes of fluid are lost.

Renal Losses. **Excessive renal losses** of potassium occur in several settings. In **metabolic alkalosis,** the intracellular potassium increases in response to the pH change. The tubular cell, however, is fooled into thinking that this potassium shift is a true potassium excess and, therefore, secretes potassium. Furthermore, as bicarbonate levels rise, eventually some bicarbonate spills into the distal tubule where it is poorly reabsorbed and, as a negatively charged ion, attracts cations, including potassium. Finally, in most conditions associated with metabolic alkalosis (e.g., vomiting), ECV depletion also is present. This stimulates aldosterone production, which acts on the distal tubule to enhance sodium reabsorption and potassium excretion.

A major cause of potassium depletion is **diuretic use.** Diuretics block sodium reabsorption in the renal tubule at sites proximal to where sodium-potassium exchange occurs. Therefore, more sodium is delivered to these sites for exchange. Furthermore, because of ECV depletion from the saline diuresis, aldosterone is stimulated, enhancing potassium secretion.

In addition to these states of secondary aldosterone stimulation, **primary hyperaldosteronism** (i.e., adrenal adenoma) also will cause potassium loss.

Renal tubular defects may result in potassium wasting, in particular the distal type of **renal tubular acidosis.** In this disorder the distal tubule is unable to secrete hydrogen ion. Therefore, as sodium is reabsorbed, only potassium is available to exchange, and excess potassium is lost.

Clinical Findings

Symptoms and Signs. The symptoms and signs of potassium depletion usually do not appear until deficiency is marked. Symptoms consist of **apathy, weakness, paresthesias, and tetany.** Irregularities of cardiac rhythm may develop. With far advanced deficiency a flaccid paralysis may occur. The cranial nerves are rarely involved, but the muscles of respiration may be so weakened that the patient has to be mechanically ventilated. Potassium depletion predisposes to **digitalis intoxication, a condition that always demands a measurement of plasma potassium.**

Laboratory Evaluation. **Determination of the plasma potassium level is the most valuable aid in the diagnosis of potassium depletion.** Diagnosis of potassium disturbances before they become severe depends on measuring the plasma level, a rather sensitive index, as shown in Figure 10–1. When hypokalemia is present **and before any therapy is given, the urinary potassium concentration is helpful in defining the etiology of depletion. If the urine potassium is less than 10 mEq/L, nonrenal losses should be suspected. When the urine potassium concentration exceeds 10 mEq/L, depletion is probably secondary to renal losses.**

The presence of metabolic alkalosis should always raise the question of potassium depletion. Gastrointestinal or renal loss of potassium or both are commonly associated with diseases producing this acid-base disorder. Despite this frequent association of potassium depletion and alkalosis, each condition does occur separately.

Changes in the electrocardiogram are not pathognomonic of potassium depletion but may be suggestive. Potassium depletion is characterized by a sagging of the ST segments, depression of the T waves, and elevation of the U waves. The Q-T interval appears to be prolonged only because the Q-U interval is mistakenly measured as the Q-T interval. Frequent **premature ventricular contractions** due to ventricular irritability also are common.

Renal concentrating ability is impaired, and tubular injury occurs in patients with chronic potassium depletion. This may result in a polyuric state with renal wasting of water.

In summary, potassium depletion may be suggested by

1. Recognition of causative events
2. Symptoms and signs of neuromuscular dysfunction
3. Electrocardiographic changes

A low plasma potassium level is confirmatory.

Prevention and Treatment

Maintenance Therapy. Because large changes in total body potassium must occur before clinically significant depletion develops, it is relatively easy to prevent potassium depletion by careful attention to maintenance therapy. **Great care in potassium administration is indicated in cases of possible renal shutdown, where there is always a danger of life-threatening potassium excess.**

Replacement Therapy. The potassium given in excess of the basic allowance constitutes **corrective therapy.** As long as a large potassium depletion exists, there is little danger in the administration of 20 mEq/hour or more, since potassium rapidly enters the cells, and significantly elevated plasma levels are not common. However, the plasma potassium is more and more easily increased as normal potassium balance is approached. For this reason, **it is not wise to completely correct potassium depletion in 1 day. Attempt to correct 30 to 50% of the calculated deficit (but not exceeding 240 mEq) in any 24 hour period, with frequent reevaluation.**

By distributing potassium dosage evenly in the fluids being administered, it usually is possible to keep potassium concentrations below 40 mEq/L in parenteral fluids. Occasionally, in cases of very severe depletion, it is necessary to use higher potassium concentrations. In such severe cases, careful control of the rate of infusion with an ECG monitor in place is mandatory to avoid a high plasma potassium concentration and cardiac standstill. Oral administration of potassium-rich foods or potassium salts is possible in patients not requiring parenteral fluids.

When potassium depletion and extracellular alkalosis coexist, potassium chloride is good treatment for both conditions. The chloride stays in the ECF, whereas the potassium may either enter cells if there is potassium depletion or be excreted in the urine in place of hydrogen.

Although oliguria usually is a contraindication to potassium therapy, uremia is not. The uremic patient often has a relatively high and fixed potassium loss, and therapy must be guided by serial measurements of the plasma potassium.

POTASSIUM EXCESS

Potassium excess usually is found in the clinical settings noted in Table 10–3.

Causes

Excessive Intake. Renal excretion normally prevents potassium excess. However, hyperkalemia can occur in a patient with normal renal function if large intravenous doses of potassium are adminstered rapidly.

TABLE 10–3. CAUSES OF POTASSIUM EXCESS (HYPERKALEMIA)

I. Excessive intake
II. Decreased renal excretion
    A. Oliguric renal failure
    B. Adrenal failure
    C. Potassium-sparing diuretics
III. Spurious hyperkalemia

Decreased Renal Excretion

Oliguric Renal Failure. When renal failure is accompanied by oliguria (a common occurrence in acute renal failure), even a normal potassium intake will exceed excretory capacity, and **potassium excess is common.** Frequently, acute renal failure is accompanied by significant tissue damage or catabolism. In either case, large amounts of potassium are released from cells. Combined with the decreased renal excretion, this often leads to life-threatening hyperkalemia.

Adrenal Failure. With the loss of adrenal mineralocorticoids (aldosterone), renal excretion of potassium is impaired, and potassium accumulates. Serum levels usually are less than 6.5 mEq/L and not hazardous. If intake is increased, however, there is a potential for much higher, dangerous levels to occur.

Potassium-sparing Diuretics. These drugs (e.g., triamterene, amiloride) are generally safe. However, when potassium-sparing diuretics are **combined with other factors that increase potassium load or reduce renal excretion,** severe hyperkalemia can occur. Risk factors for this complication include decreased renal function, increased potassium intake, or the new class of antihypertensives known as converting enzyme inhibitors. These agents block the conversion of angiotensin I to angiotensin II, resulting in loss of angiotensin's effect on the adrenal—the production of aldosterone. As with primary aldosterone deficiency, renal retention of potassium will occur.

Spurious Hyperkalemia. Occasionally, hyperkalemia is due to spurious factors and is not indicative of potassium excess. This occurs when **hemolysis or thrombocytosis** is present in the blood specimen before assay. With **hemolysis,** the red blood cell potassium leaks into the serum, giving an erroneous measurement. In **thrombocytosis,** the large number of platelets present leak potassium into the serum during clotting of the laboratory specimen. Careful collection of blood should prevent hemolysis, and prevention of clotting with heparin will allow correct plasma potassium assays in these patients.

Clinical Findings

Symptoms and Signs. Signs and symptoms of potassium excess **seldom occur.** Occasionally, a patient will develop weakness and even a flaccid type of paralysis that is indistinguishable from that seen with hypokalemia.

Laboratory Evaluation. Laboratory evaluation **begins and ends with the electrocardiogram (ECG).** What is crucial is the effect of potassium on cell depolarization, which the ECG reflects. Because other factors (e.g., calcium concentration, sodium concentration) also influence depolarization, the serum potassium determination is of much less value than the ECG itself (Fig.10–3).

The earliest ECG signs of potassium intoxication are the T wave changes of

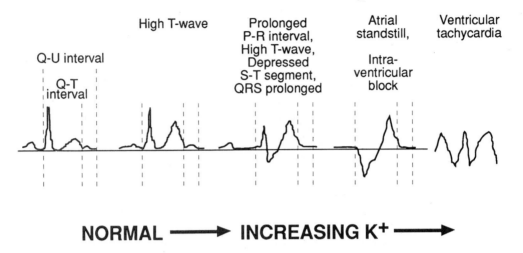

Figure 10–3. Changes in electrocardiogram with increasing hyperkalemia.

tenting (the usual asymmetrical T wave becomes symmetrical) and heightening. Next P-R prolongation occurs, followed by QRS widening. This is an important change and often heralds rapid deterioration to atrioventricular block and ventricular fibrillation.

Usually, **serious ECG changes are seen with plasma potassium levels above 7 mEq/L and fibrillation at levels above 8.** With severe hypocalcemia, however, plasma potassium levels below 6 may prove fatal. On the other hand, with a calcium of 12 mEq/L, a plasma potassium of 8 can be accompanied by a normal ECG.

Hyperkalemia in states of potassium excess may be markedly aggravated by a reduction in blood pH. With marked acidosis, a plasma potassium level of 6 to 7 mEq/L may reflect normal intracellular stores, or a normal plasma potassium may reflect depleted stores.

Treatment
Potassium intoxication represents a medical emergency that can lead to the death of the patient from cardiac arrest. The specific measures used to treat hyperkalemia are listed in Table 10–4.

Conservative Measures. **Calcium chloride should be used if there is QRS widening or more severe ECG changes.** Ten milliliters of a 10% solution should be infused over 1 to 2 minutes while observing the ECG. When the QRS is of normal width, the rapid infusion of calcium can be stopped. The calcium level is then maintained by diluting 20 to 30 mL of 10% calcium chloride in 500 mL of D_5W (5% dextrose in water) and infusing this over 6 hours. Calcium chloride is preferable to other calcium salts because of the much larger amount of elemental calcium availa-

TABLE 10–4. TREATMENT OF HYPERKALEMIA

Therapy	Onset of Action	Duration of Action
Calcium infusion	1 min	5–60 min
Slower acting agents		
Glucose and insulin	15–30 min	4–8 hours
Sodium bicarbonate	15–30 min	4–8 hours
Cation exchange resins		
Rectal	30–90 min	Indefinite (repeat)
Oral	2–12 hours	Indefinite (repeat)
Dialysis	Immediate	Indefinite (repeat)

ble compared to other preparations. Calcium acts at the cell membrane to oppose the effects of high potassium.

The slower acting approaches can then be used to lower potassium until the primary problem is corrected or dialysis is started. These include **glucose** and **insulin**, and **bicarbonate** (which drive potassium into cells) and **resins** (which exchange potassium for another cation in the gut).

Dialysis. If available, dialysis will immediately lower the serum potassium level. An emergency peritoneal dialysis can be performed by infusing through a Y connection 1 L of 5% D & S (5% dextrose in normal saline) and 1 L of 1/6 mol/L sodium lactate. Leave these 2 L in the peritoneal space for 20 to 30 minutes and then drain and repeat the cycle if necessary.

There are special considerations for chronic dialysis patients with hyperkalemia. Occasionally, otherwise healthy chronic dialysis patients will develop dangerous potassium intoxication. Since their liver glycogen stores and acid-base balance are normal, intravenous glucose and sodium bicarbonate are relatively ineffective. Immediate dialysis is mandatory. Calcium infusion should be held in reserve as the last line of defense and, once started, should be continued with ECG monitoring until dialysis is well underway.

STUDY CASES

Case 1

History. A 72-year-old man was hospitalized for weakness and confusion. Three days previously, he had developed severe diarrhea with stools described as resembling egg whites. There was a history of two similar, although less severe, episodes in the preceding 2 months. He had not vomited and had taken fluids liberally because of thirst.

Physical Examination. The admission physical examination revealed an acutely ill, apathetic elderly man. Blood pressure was 110/70 recumbent, 90/50 sitting. Pulse was 80/minute recumbent, 100/minute sitting. Respirations were 23/minute. Weight was 66 kg (usual 66 kg). The neck veins were flat, skin turgor was poor, and oral mucous membranes were slightly dry. Heart and lungs were normal. No abdominal masses or tenderness was present, and the bowel sounds were hypoactive. The prostate and rectum were normal, and stool guaiac was 1+. There was no edema, and the neurologic examination was normal except for hypoactive deep tendon reflexes.

Laboratory Data. Hct 54%., WBC 16,000. Serum sodium 119, potassium 2.3, chloride 85, bicarbonate 22 mEq/L, urea nitrogen 78, glucose 115, creatinine 4.2 mg/dL. Arterial blood: pH 7.38, P_{CO_2} 38. U/A: electrolytes Na^+ 15, K^+ 12, Cl^- 19 mEq/L. Stool electrolytes: Na^+ 120, K^+ 50 mEq/L. Stool volume 500 mL in 8 hours.

1. Discuss the disorders of fluid and electrolyte balance and their pathogenesis.
2. Quantitate the degree of each fluid/electrolyte disorder noted.
3. What are the physical manifestations of the fluid and electrolyte disorders noted?
4. Outline a plan of therapy in the worksheet.

BASIC ALLOWANCE

	Volume	Na+	K+	H+	Cl-	HCO3-
Urine				▨		▨
S + I		▨	▨	▨		▨
GI						
TOTAL:						

DIAGNOSES:
1. ECV (Saline)
2. Water
3. Acid/Base
4. Potassium

Corrections	Volume	Na+	K+	H+	Cl-	HCO3-
Saline +/-			▨	▨		▨
Water +/-		▨	▨	▨		▨
Acid/Base +/-						
Potassium +/-	▨	▨				
SUM: Basics + Corrections						

Case 2

History. A 45-year-old farmer was involved in a tractor accident 32 hours previously that fractured his left femur and severely contused his right leg. At the time you receive this information, he has arrived in the emergency room and is being evaluated by an orthopedic surgeon.

Physical Examination. Temperature 36.3°C, pulse 110, respirations 22, blood pressure 80/50 supine. An ECG was obtained just before your arrival (Fig.10–4).

5. In view of the history and ECG, what is the most likely fluid and electrolyte problem?
6. What is the etiology of this problem?
7. What single drug would be the most useful in immediately reversing the ECG abnormalities? How long would you expect this effect to persist?
8. What other forms of therapy would you also consider for short-term (2 to 4 hours) treatment of this fluid and electrolyte problem? Explain the advantages and disadvantages of each potential treatment.

Course. After correction of hypotension and other treatment, the patient was found to be oliguric (12 mL urine hourly). The following laboratory data became available: Hct 41%, WBC 15,000, serum sodium 138, chloride 101, bicarbonate 22 mEq/L; glucose 110, urea nitrogen 24, creatinine 1.6 mg/dL, potassium 5.5 mEq/L. U/A: 310 mOsm/

V_2 Lead

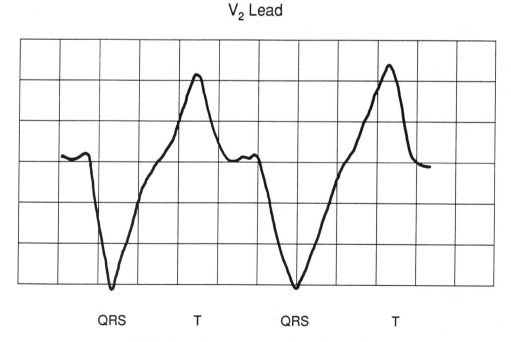

QRS   T   QRS   T

Figure 10–4. Electrocardiogram (V_2 lead) from Case 2.

BASIC ALLOWANCE

	Volume	Na+	K+	H+	Cl-	HCO3-
Urine						
S + I						
GI						
TOTAL:						

DIAGNOSES:
1. ECV (Saline)
2. Water
3. Acid/Base
4. Potassium

Corrections	Volume	Na+	K+	H+	Cl-	HCO3-
Saline +/-						
Water +/-						
Acid/Base +/-						
Potassium +/-						
SUM: Basics + Corrections						

L, pH 5, protein, glucose, ketones negative, occult blood positive, sediment showed a few tubular cells. Urine sodium 40 mEq/L, creatinine 10 mg/dL.

9. Explain the significance of these data in treating the patient.
10. Plan treatment using the worksheet.

Case 3

History. This 48-year-old man has a long history of peptic ulcer and recently began to vomit frequently. X-ray studies demonstrated pyloric obstruction.

Physical Examination. Weight 94 kg (usual 94 kg), temperature 37°C, respirations 14, pulse 84, blood pressure 140/80 supine and 110/65 sitting. Because of obesity, neck veins were not visible.

Laboratory Data. Hct 38%, serum sodium 130, potassium 2.8, chloride 76, glucose 82, urea nitrogen 12, creatinine 1.1 mg/dL. U/A: unremarkable. Arterial blood gases: pH 7.51, P_{CO_2} 55, P_{O_2} 85. Fluid balance for the past 24 hours is as follows:

	Input	**Output**
Volume	4000 mL	2600 mL urine
Sodium	300 mEq	1000 mL S & I
Potassium	80 mEq	1800 mL GI
Cl⁻	380 mEq	5400 mL total

BASIC ALLOWANCE	Volume	Na+	K+	H+	Cl-	HCO3-
Urine						
S + I						
GI						
TOTAL:						

DIAGNOSES:
1. ECV (Saline)
2. Water
3. Acid/Base
4. Potassium

Corrections	Volume	Na+	K+	H+	Cl-	HCO3-
Saline +/-						
Water +/-						
Acid/Base +/-						
Potassium +/-						
SUM: Basics + Corrections						

11. What fluid and electrolyte problems are present?
12. Explain the pathogenesis of the arterial blood abnormalities.
13. What is the significance, if any, of the lack of weight change?
14. Estimate the urine electrolytes.
15. Plan treatment for the next 24 hours using the worksheet.

ANSWERS TO STUDY CASES

Case 1

1. **Discuss the disorders of fluid and electrolyte balance and their pathogenesis.**
2. **Quantitate the degree of each fluid/electrolyte disorder noted.**
3. **What are the physical manifestations of the fluid and electrolyte disorders noted?**

Water. The marked hyponatremia (119 mEq/L) documents significant water excess and is probably the cause of his confusional state. In a patient weighing 66 kg normally, this represents approximately a 6 L excess of total body water. With the presence of azotemia and extracellular volume depletion, it is likely that this problem was produced by an oral intake in excess of renal excretory capacity. It is also possible that acute volume depletion stimulated ADH release, with renal conservation of water. The lack of a highly concentrated urine does not eliminate this supposition in the presence of this degree of azotemia.

ECV. Several factors, such as the history of marked diarrhea, flat neck veins, postural hypotension, and an elevated hematocrit, point to depletion. The absence of a prior history of renal disease and a normal appearing urinalysis suggest that renal insufficiency may be due to a marked reduction in renal blood flow. The lack of weight change should not detract from the diagnosis, since the patient has marked water excess. Assuming that the patient has ingested adequate calories and has not lost anhydrous tissue mass, the following calculation indicates that he has indeed lost 20 to 25% of his ECV.

$$\frac{\text{Plasma volume}}{\text{change}} = \frac{\text{current Hct} - \text{initial Hct}}{\text{initial Hct}} = \frac{54-45}{45} = 20\%$$

$$\text{Body weight} = \Delta \text{ECV} + \Delta \text{ICV}$$

$$0 \text{ kg} = \Delta \text{ECV} + (0.4 \times 66) \left(\frac{139-119}{139} \right)$$

$$\Delta \text{ECV} = -3.8 \text{ L}$$

This is a substantial ECV deficit. If water excess were not present, it would be even greater, since about one third of the excess water is in the ECV. If the water excess alone were completely corrected, the ECV would decline by approximately 2 L. Thus, the true saline or ECV deficit is over 5.0 L.

Acid-Base. Although it might be expected that metabolic acidosis could result from a large loss of bicarbonate-rich fluid from the lower colon, the arterial pH and serum bicarbonate suggest no abnormal acid-base problems.

Potassium. In the absence of an acid-base disturbance, the severe hypokalemia is consistent with a marked depletion of total body potassium. The potassium nomogram (Fig. 10–1) would suggest approximately 20% depletion, or a loss of 500 to 600 mEq. It is likely that this depletion has been from the gastrointestinal tract in view of the quantity of potassium lost in his colonic fluid. Potassium depletion in this patient is reflected in his weakness and hyporeflexia.

Clinical Diagnosis. In view of the rapid onset of severe diarrhea, bacterial causes as well as ulcerative and granulomatous colitis must always be considered. The history of prior but less severe episodes in the preceding 2 months and the description of the stool specimens as "resembling egg whites" suggests the likelihood of an unusual lesion. A villous adenoma was found in this patient on sigmoidoscopy.

4. Outline a plan of therapy.

A possible plan for treatment is shown on the accompanying fluid balance worksheet 10–1. Basic allowance includes gastrointestinal fluid replacement for ongoing colonic losses. Enough water is removed from the overall plan to

BASIC ALLOWANCE

	Volume	Na+	K+	H+	Cl-	HCO3-
Urine	1500	50	40		90	
S + I	1000					
GI	1500	180	75		255	
TOTAL:	4000	230	115		345	

DIAGNOSES:
1. ECV (Saline) DEPLETION
2. Water EXCESS
3. Acid/Base SATISFACTORY (not necessary to treat)
4. Potassium DEPLETION

Corrections	Volume	Na+	K+	H+	Cl-	HCO3-
Saline +/-	+3000	450			450	
Water +/-	-2000					
Acid/Base +/-						
Potassium +/-			85		85	
SUM: Basics + Corrections	5000	680	200		880	

Worksheet 10–1. Fluid balance worksheet, Case 1, answers.

produce isotonic saline replacement. Supplemental potassium is added to start repletion.

Comment on Therapy. It might be useful to give more potassium. However, unless it is an emergency, giving more than 40 mEq KCl in each liter is considered hazardous. Therefore, we have arbitrarily added an 85 mEq correction, so that we give a maximum safe potassium dose in the 5 L this patient will receive. Should a patient require such high doses (as, for instance, if the rate of loss is very great), continuous ECG monitoring would be needed.

Case 2

5. In view of the history and ECG, what is the most likely fluid and electrolyte problem?

The history, physical examination, and ECG suggest hypovolemic shock and hyperkalemia with cardiotoxicity (note the absence of P waves and tenting of T waves).

6. What is the etiology of this problem?

The trauma to large muscles produces cellular disruption and release of intracellular contents, including large amounts of potassium and myoglobin. The latter substance is nephrotoxic, particularly in the setting of renal hypoperfusion and high titers of catecholamines secondary to the hypotension that resulted from blood loss into the injured tissues. The rapid release of potassium into the ECF plus some metabolic acidosis, as a result of hypotension and poor renal excretion, impede cellular uptake and renal excretion.

7. What single drug would be the most useful in immediately reversing the ECG abnormalities? How long would you expect this effect to persist?

The ECG changes can be reversed by intravenous calcium (5 to 15 mg/kg) given as small bolus injections. The duration of effect of each bolus may be quite short (30 to 60 minutes) but will prevent cardiac arrest and allow time to start other measures for removing potassium from the ECF.

8. What other forms of therapy would you also consider for short-term (2 to 4 hours) treatment of this fluid and electrolyte problem? Explain the advantages and disadvantages of each potential treatment.

Glucose produces potassium transport into viable cells. It is effective only if the glucose load causes release of insulin and the formation of intracellular substrates that can bind potassium. It often is given with exogenous insulin, although this is not necessary except in diabetic patients. *Advantage*: Readily convenient therapy. *Disadvantage*: May produce hyperglycemia and intracellular contraction if overdose occurs.

Sodium bicarbonate. By correcting metabolic acidosis or causing a mild alkalosis, potassium is shifted into viable cells. *Advantage*: Readily available therapy. *Disadvantage*: Too vigorous therapy will produce marked ECF expansion. If hypertonic solution is used (1000 mEq/L), cellular contraction and hyperosmolarity are produced.

Kayexalate. This oral cation exchange resin will bind potassium in the gut and reduce the ECF concentration. *Advantage*: Commonly available. *Disadvantage*: Works slowly over hours to days; may cause fecal impaction if not given with a purgative; must be given rectally if patient unable to take orally.

9. Explain the significance of these data in treating the patient.

The finding of persistent oliguria despite correction of the ECF deficit and hypotension is a sign usually indicating renal injury and acute renal failure (ARF). The urine osmolarity and the U/P osmolar ratio of about 1 are compatible with ARF. Finally, the fractional excretion of sodium (FE_{Na}) is greater than 1, a finding also suggesting ARF as opposed to a diagnosis of prerenal azotemia.

BASIC ALLOWANCE

	Volume	Na+	K+	H+	Cl-	HCO3-
Urine	250	8	7	▨	15	▨
S + I	1000	▨	▨	▨	▨	▨
GI						
TOTAL:						

DIAGNOSES:
1. ECV (Saline) NORMAL
2. Water NORMAL
3. Acid/Base MILD ACIDOSIS
4. Potassium MILD HYPERKALEMIA

Corrections	Volume	Na+	K+	H+	Cl-	HCO3-
Saline +/-		-8	▨		-8	▨
Water +/-		▨	▨		▨	▨
Acid/Base +/-						
Potassium +/-	▨		-7		-7	
SUM: Basics + Corrections	1250	0	0	0	0	

Worksheet 10–2. Fluid balance worksheet, Case 2, answers.

10. Plan treatment.

The diagnosis of ARF indicates that conservative fluid management is indicated to prevent fluid overload. Plans for dialysis as indicated for severe hypervolemia, hyperkalemia, or acidosis are made. Reductions in all drugs requiring renal elimination are made. A possible plan for treatment at this time is shown on fluid balance worksheet 10–2.

Case 3

11. What fluid and electrolyte problems are present?

ECF. Some depletion is evidenced by orthostatic blood pressure changes. Since intravascular volume must be decreased by at least 750 mL (15%) to account for this, total ECV should be down at least 3000 mL.

Water. Serum sodium concentration is low. In view of normal serum glucose, the hyponatremia reflects cellular swelling and a state of relative water excess of at least 3 L.

Acid-base. The history of gastric fluid loss plus an elevated serum bicarbonate and arterial pH are all compatible with metabolic alkalosis. The P_{CO_2} is increased because of adaptive hypoventilation. The anion gap is normal. There is, thus, no evidence of other significant acid-base disorders.

Potassium. The serum level is low and is partially corrected by adjustments for the arterial pH. However, the low corrected value reflects a total body depletion of about 10% or 400 mEq.

12. Explain the pathogenesis of the arterial blood abnormalities.

This topic is discussed in Chapter 11. The problem is initiated by loss of hydrochloric acid in gastric fluid. The loss of hydrion causes an alkalosis, and the chloride depletion prevents the kidney from excreting bicarbonate. The high P_{CO_2} is caused by the alkalosis depressing the respiratory center. Despite hypoventilation, however, oxygen exchange is adequate. Sodium chloride loss also stimulates aldosterone production, which further aggravates the situation.

13. What is the significance, if any, of the lack of weight change?

The lack of weight change appears to be explained by a loss of isotonic fluid from vomiting plus a gain of solute-free water.

14. Estimate the urine electrolytes.

Because of hypovolemia with secondary aldosteronism, urine sodium and chloride would be low and potassium moderately high. Urine pH and HCO_3 would be hard to predict, but aciduria with low HCO_3 is possible.

15. Plan treatment for the next 24 hours.

The problems noted can be corrected by administration of sodium and potassium chloride. See the fluid balance worksheet 10–3 for a possible approach. This type of problem may be ameliorated in part also by the use of cimetidine, an H_2-antagonist. Cimetidine reduces the hydrochloric acid production and, hence, the loss that occurs when nasogastric suction is used as a part of medical therapy for pyloric obstruction.

BASIC ALLOWANCE

	Volume	Na+	K+	H+	Cl-	HCO3-
Urine	1500	50	40	▨	90	▨
S + I	1000	▨	▨	▨	▨	▨
GI	1800	180	18		198	
TOTAL:	4300	230	58		288	

DIAGNOSES:
1. ECV (Saline) DEPLETION
2. Water EXCESS
3. Acid/Base METABOLIC ALKALOSIS
4. Potassium DEPLETION

Corrections	Volume	Na+	K+	H+	Cl-	HCO3-
Saline +/-	+3000	+450	▨		+450	▨
Water +/-	-1000	▨	▨		▨	▨
Acid/Base +/-						
Potassium +/-	▨		+100		+100	
SUM: Basics + Corrections	6300	680	158	0	838	

IV Orders:

Worksheet 10–3. Fluid balance worksheet, Case 3, answers.

Acid-Base

INTRODUCTION

To maintain normal physiology, the body regulates levels of numerous substances within narrow limits. These limits exist so that biochemical processes, which require a specific, stable milieu, can continue their life-sustaining roles. Perhaps most tightly regulated of these substances is the hydrogen ion. This chapter considers how acid-base regulation occurs and how the four primary abnormalities (metabolic acidosis, metabolic alkalosis, respiratory acidosis, and respiratory alkalosis) develop. Since this is a renal text and renal problems lead to metabolic abnormalities, primary emphasis is on the metabolic acid-base disorders.

STUDY OBJECTIVES

To understand the

1. Causes
2. Diagnosis
3. Management

of the primary acid-base disorders

1. Metabolic acidosis
2. Metabolic alkalosis
3. Respiratory acidosis
4. Respiratory alkalosis

PHYSIOLOGY AND PATHOPHYSIOLOGY

Acid-Base Regulation
The body attempts to maintain a pH between 7.35 and 7.43 (hydrogen ion concentration between 35 and 45 nmol/L). This is achieved despite considerable variation in acid-base intake. With normal diet and metabolism, many **thousands of milliequivalents of volatile hydrogen ion are eliminated by the lungs as CO_2** based on the reaction

$$H^+ + HCO_3^- \leftrightarrow H_2CO_3 \leftrightarrow CO_2 + H_2O$$

The great majority of hydrogen ion is eliminated by this route.

A relatively small amount of nonvolatile acids, 70 to 100 mEq daily, also is generated from a variety of sources, and these must be eliminated as well. The major sources are shown in Table 11–1. These acids are **not metabolized to CO_2 and cannot be excreted by the lungs.** The only other route of elimination, the kidneys, must be used.

I. **Sources of metabolic (nonvolatile) acid.**
   A. **Diet.** With a typical diet, about 30 mEq of hydrogen ion (acid) is added to the body daily. With a **very high animal protein intake,** this can be increased markedly. On the other hand, the diet consumed by herbivores and human vegetarians may be neutral or actually alkaline.
   B. **Incomplete metabolism.** Normally, incomplete metabolism of glucose and other carbohydrates results in about 30 mEq daily of **ketoacids, beta-hydroxybutyrate,** and similar acidic substances, which require renal excretion.
   C. **Stool loss of bicarbonate.** Around 20 mEq of HCO_3^- is lost in the stools daily. From the acid-base perspective, **loss of bicarbonate leaves a hydrogen ion free to increase the acid load.** Thus, loss of HCO_3^- is equivalent to adding the same amount of acid to the body.

II. **Elimination of acid-base.**
   A. **Lungs.** The lungs eliminate a large amount of volatile acid as CO_2 (20,000 mmol/day). **This can be greatly increased or modestly decreased if the lungs are normal** and acid-base receptors perceive a need for such alterations.

TABLE 11–1. SOURCES AND AMOUNTS OF NONVOLATILE ACIDS

Source	Amount/day
Diet	30 mEq
Incomplete metabolism of organic acids	30 mEq
Stool bicarbonate loss	20 mEq

B. **Kidneys.**
  i. **Acid excretion. Normally, the kidneys are called on to excrete 70 to 100 mEq of acid daily. This can be reduced to zero or increased three- to fourfold if necessary.**
  ii. **Alkali excretion. If faced with an alkaline load, the kidneys can excrete many hundreds of milliequivalents of bicarbonate.** Theoretically, more than 1000 mEq of bicarbonate could be excreted daily, but such large excretion rates are rarely if ever seen.

Abnormal States

Lungs. Abnormalities of pulmonary function can lead to **reduced CO_2 levels (increased ventilation) or too much CO_2 (reduced ventilation).** The alkalosis or acidosis, respectively, that results is obviously a consequence of the shift in the carbonic acid buffering system.

Kidneys. A variety of renal lesions or abnormalities of various hormones can lead to deficient or excess hydrogen ion excretion, excess bicarbonate loss, or excess bicarbonate regeneration, with various effects on the acid-base status.

Metabolic Abnormalities. **Diabetes, out of control,** results in a marked increase in incomplete metabolism of carbohydrates, with a resultant acidosis (diabetic ketoacidosis). With poor tissue perfusion (**shock**), anaerobic metabolism leads to a marked increase in lactic acid generation and **lactic acidosis.** There are other metabolic disorders that also may lead to excess acids of these sorts, but diabetic ketoacidosis and lactic acidosis are the most common.

Gastrointestinal Abnormalities. Excessive gastric acid may be produced and lost (e.g., protracted **vomiting**), with resultant alkalosis. Other intestinal secretions, such as **diarrhea** fluid, usually contain large amounts of bicarbonate. Metabolic acidosis occurs with significant loss of these fluids.

DATABASE AND OTHER CONSIDERATIONS

Measurements and Calculations

The acid-base status of the body is evaluated by measuring the **hydrogen concentration, serum bicarbonate (HCO_3^-), pCO_2, and the anion gap (AG).** To understand the body's buffer system, one must be familiar with the **Henderson-Hasselbalch equation.** Because all body buffer systems are in equilibrium with the same concentration of hydrogen ion (isohydric principle, see Chapter 8), the acid-base status can be expressed by measuring changes in any of the body buffer systems. Clinically, **the carbonic acid-bicarbonate system is most important.** By applying the law of mass action to the following reaction

$$CO_2 + H_2O \leftrightarrow H_2CO_3 \leftrightarrow H^+ + HCO_3^-$$

one obtains the classic Henderson-Hasselbalch equation

$$pH = 6.1 + \log \frac{[HCO_3^-]}{P_{CO_2}}$$

Many physicians find this equation cumbersome and prefer the same expression without the logarithms.

$$[H^+] = 24 \times \frac{P_{CO_2}}{[HCO_3^-]}$$

Where H^+ = hydrogen ion concentration in nmol/L
  P_{CO_2} = partial pressure of CO_2 in mm Hg
  HCO_3^- = bicarbonate concentration in mEq/L
  Normally, pH is 7.40, $[HCO_3^-]$ is 24, $[H^+]$ is 40, and P_{CO_2} is 40.

Since clinical results are expressed as the P_{CO_2} and $[HCO_3^-]$, it is easy to calculate the $[H^+]$. This can then be converted to pH by taking the negative logarithm or by using Table 11–2.

The pH of blood (or any other fluid compartment of the body), therefore, can be determined from the concentration of bicarbonate and P_{CO_2} (carbonic acid) present. Thus, a change in blood pH must be accompanied by a change in one or both of these variables. It is important to note also that it is the ratio of bicarbonate to carbonic acid and not the absolute value of either one that defines the pH of the patient. Therefore, to evaluate a patient's acid-base status, two of the three variables (pH, P_{CO_2}, and bicarbonate) must be known.

TABLE 11–2. Relationship of pH to H^+ Concentration

H+	pH
158	6.8
126	6.9
100	7.0
79	7.1
63	7.2
50	7.3
40	7.4
32	7.5
25	7.6
20	7.7
15.8	7.8
12.6	7.9

Specific Disturbances

When the arterial blood pH is less than 7.4 (H^+ greater than 40), the patient has acidosis. When the pH is greater than 7.4, the patient has alkalosis. Acidosis can be caused by an increase in Pco_2 or a decrease in bicarbonate. Conversely, alkalosis can be caused by a decrease in Pco_2 or an increase in bicarbonate. Since Pco_2 is determined by the lungs, disorders of pH caused primarily by abnormalities in Pco_2 are called respiratory acidosis and respiratory alkalosis. Disorders that result in abnormal bicarbonate concentrations are termed metabolic. Thus, **four primary acid-base disturbances are recognized.**

1. **Metabolic acidosis is associated with a fall in plasma pH and a decrease in plasma bicarbonate.** This disorder may arise from removal of bicarbonate from the body in alkaline fluids or by addition of hydrion, which reacts with bicarbonate to form CO_2 and H_2O.
2. **Metabolic alkalosis, similarly, is associated with a rise in pH and an increase in plasma bicarbonate and usually is caused by loss of HCl** through vomiting or gastric secretion.
3. **Respiratory acidosis is associated with a fall in pH resulting from a primary increase in Pco_2 due to primary hypoventilation.**
4. **Respiratory alkalosis is associated with a rise in pH from a decrease in Pco_2 due to hyperventilation.**

Compensation

The body tries to correct (compensate for) each of the primary acid-base disturbances.

Metabolic Disorders. **With metabolic acidosis or alkalosis, the pulmonary response will attempt to correct the pH.** Thus, with metabolic acidosis, hyperventilation will decrease the Pco_2 and reduce the H^+ concentration. With metabolic alkalosis, hypoventilation will occur, the Pco_2 will rise, and the H^+ concentration will return toward normal. Respiratory compensation for alkalosis is limited because hypoxia (low Po_2) develops with decreasing ventilation, and the hypoxic stimulus to breathe eventually will override the alkalotic inhibition of ventilation (usually at a Po_2 of around 60 mm Hg). **Respiratory compensation occurs immediately.**

Respiratory Disorders. With respiratory acid-base disorders, **the kidneys compensate by regulating bicarbonate levels.** Increasing production and retention (thus raising the bicarbonate) in respiratory acidosis or excreting more bicarbonate and lowering the plasma level in alkalosis both serve to protect the pH. With acute respiratory disorders, minimal bicarbonate compensation occurs (because **it takes several hours for the kidneys to respond**). With chronic respiratory disorders, on the other hand, marked bicarbonate changes occur. Table 11–3 depicts the compensatory changes expected in the various disorders.

TABLE 11–3. ACID-BASE COMPENSATION BY LUNGS OR KIDNEY

Disorder	Expected Compensation
Metabolic acidosis	For each 1 mEq fall in HCO_3^-, P_{CO_2} declines 1–1.3 mm Hg
Metabolic alkalosis	For each 1 mEq rise in HCO_3^-, P_{CO_2} rises 0.6 mm Hg[a]
Acute respiratory acidosis	For each 1 mm rise in P_{CO_2}, HCO_3^- rises 0.1 mEq
Acute respiratory alkalosis	For each 1 mm fall in P_{CO_2}, HCO_3^- falls 0.2 mEq
Chronic respiratory acidosis	For each 1 mm rise in P_{CO_2}, HCO_3^- rises 0.35 mEq
Chronic respiratory alkalosis	For each 1 mm fall in P_{CO_2}, HCO_3^- falls 0.5 mEq

[a]Remember, hypoxia limits this response.

Incomplete Compensation. **When the expected compensation fails to occur, it is because of disease in that system.** This is then termed a **mixed or combined disorder.** For instance, if the bicarbonate drops to 15 mEq/L and the P_{CO_2} does not fall below 40 mm Hg, a much more severe acidosis results because of both a metabolic and a respiratory problem. This would be termed a **combined metabolic and respiratory acidosis.** A metabolic disorder could similarly be identified as accompanying a respiratory disorder if the kidneys failed to adjust the bicarbonate adequately.

Anion Gap

Cations (positively charged ions) are equal in number to anions in the body. **In the bloodstream, where the electrolytes are measured, cations seem to exceed anions in number.** This difference, the anion deficit or anion gap (AG), normally is **accounted for by plasma proteins and usually amounts to about 10 to 12 mEq/L** (Fig. 11–1). Although the AG can be determined by precisely calculating all the cations and anions, it is sufficient to determine just the sodium, bicarbonate, and chloride. The remaining anions are almost always equal in amount to the remaining cations. Therefore, the **AG traditionally is defined as the difference between the major cation, sodium, and the major anions, chloride plus bicarbonate.**

$$\text{Anion gap} = Na^+ - (Cl^- + HCO_3^-)$$

Of what use is this fact? **First, an increased AG always means a metabolic acidosis is present. Second, an increased AG implies that the cause of the acidosis must be retention of some acid other than HCl.** This is discussed further in the next section.

Acid-Base Nomogram

Appropriate management of pH problems usually requires measurement of pH, P_{CO_2}, and HCO_3^- concentrations. Once these values are known, assessing them with an acid-base nomogram often will be helpful (Fig. 11–2). The shaded areas in the nomogram show the range of values generally found with each disorder.

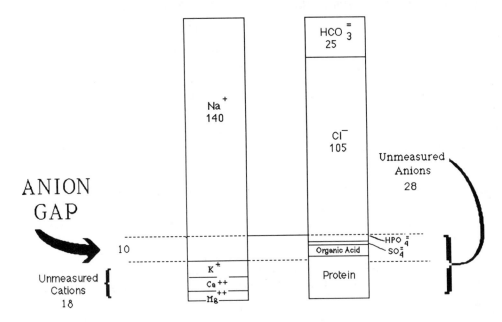

Figure 11–1. The anion gap.

These ranges assume that respiratory compensation has had time to occur in the metabolic disorders and that metabolic compensation has occurred in response to the chronic respiratory disorders. It is assumed that compensation has not had time to occur in the acute respiratory disorders. Values that fall within the shaded areas (Fig. 11–2) usually represent a simple disorder. Values that fall outside these areas can represent combined disorders, disorders in transition (e.g., from acute to chronic respiratory acidosis), or technical and laboratory errors. Use of the nomogram facilitates understanding of acid-base disorders.

METABOLIC ACIDOSIS

Causes
Metabolic acidosis results from three types of disorders: excess acid load, decreased acid excretion by the kidney, or alkali (bicarbonate) loss. With an excess acid load or decreased acid excretion, either an increased or normal AG can be seen. With bicarbonate loss, chloride is retained and the AG is unchanged (Fig. 11–3).

What determines whether an AG develops in metabolic acidosis? Whenever hydrogen ion (acid) is added to the system, bicarbonate is consumed. Hydrogen ion, a cation, cannot be added without an anion. For each molecule of bicarbonate

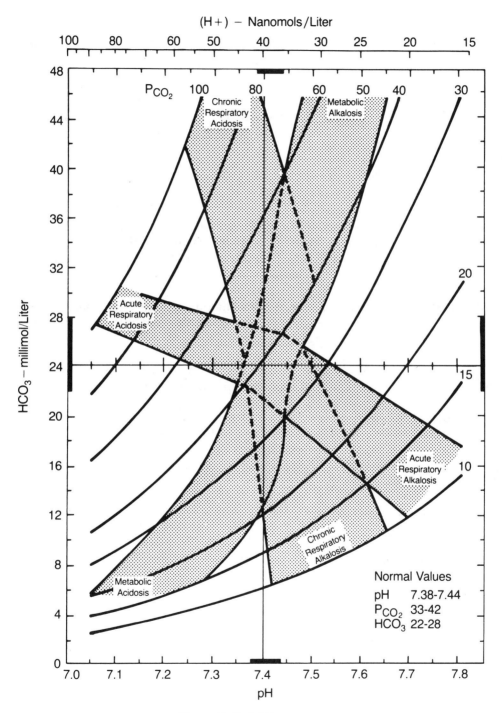

Figure 11–2. Acid-base nomogram.

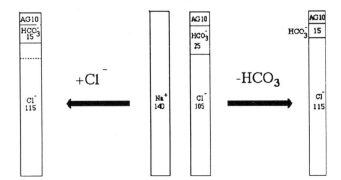

Figure 11–3. Metabolic acidosis with a normal anion gap.

consumed, a negative charge of some other type (which was given with the hydrogen ion) is added to the body fluids. **If the negatively charged ion happens to be chloride, no increase in AG will develop. If it is any other anion, the AG will be increased.**

Normal Anion Gap. In what situations does chloride replace bicarbonate in metabolic acidosis (this is sometimes known as **hyperchloremic metabolic acidosis**)? This occurs in three basic settings (Table 11–4).

Addition of HCl (or NH₄Cl) to Body Fluids. These acids can be administered intravenously as part of parenteral nutrition therapy or to correct alkalosis.

Loss of Bicarbonate. With **diarrhea** or with some enteric fistulas, large amounts of bicarbonate may be lost. Chloride is then retained as replacement. **In renal tubular acidosis,** due to a defect in **proximal** tubular cell function, bicarbonate is lost in the urine. As a consequence, chloride is reabsorbed in larger quantities than usual.

TABLE 11–4. CAUSES OF METABOLIC ACIDOSIS

I. Normal anion gap (hyperchloremic metabolic acidosis)
  A. Excess intake (HCl, NH₄Cl)
  B. Bicarbonate loss
    1. GI tract
      a. Diarrhea
      b. Fistulas
    2. Proximal renal tubular acidosis
  C. Decreased renal acid secretion (distal renal tubular acidosis)
II. Increased anion gap
  A. Ketoacidosis
    1. Diabetes mellitus
    2. Alcohol
  B. Lactic acidosis (usually due to shock)
  C. Poisons
  D. Renal failure

Decreased Renal Acid Excretion. **In the distal types of renal tubular acidosis,** HCl is not excreted adequately. The hydrogen ion retention leads to bicarbonate consumption, and the chloride again replaces the bicarbonate. In addition, in the distal types of acidosis, bicarbonate regeneration (see Chapter 8) also is defective, further contributing to the bicarbonate deficit. Again, chloride is retained by the renal tubule in place of the absent bicarbonate.

Increased Anion Gap. In metabolic acidosis with an increased AG, **the acid that accumulates is associated with an anion other than chloride.** There are four general conditions in which high AG metabolic acidosis occurs (Table 11–4).

Ketoacidosis. In **diabetes mellitus** when there is inadequate insulin effect, carbohydrates are incompletely metabolized. A number of ketoacids then accumulate and result in an increased AG. **Alcohol** occasionally interferes with carbohydrate metabolism and leads to ketoacidosis.

Lactic Acidosis. Lactic acid accumulates dramatically when tissues must function with markedly decreased oxygen consumption (i.e., in an anaerobic state). This may occur with generalized **circulatory insufficiency** (e.g., cardiac arrest, septic shock), when large volumes of tissue are ischemic or infarcted, or in **severe hypoxia from any cause.**

Poisons or Overdose. Perhaps the most common cause in this category is **aspirin overdose**, with the salicylate anion increasing the AG. Other toxins, such as **ethylene glycol (antifreeze)**, may be inappropriately consumed, leading to AG acidosis as well.

Renal Failure. In total renal failure, anions of other acids (sulfuric, phosphoric) also are retained, with an increase in the AG. This contrasts with renal tubular acidosis, in which HCl accumulates and HCO_3^- is lost.

Diagnosis and Workup

In most patients, clinical signs and symptoms are not dramatic. Only occasionally is metabolic acidosis suspected from the moment a patient is seen. Therefore, metabolic acidosis usually is not a concern until the laboratory reports a **low bicarbonate level.**

Evaluation of Bicarbonate Level. The evaluation of metabolic acidosis then becomes the evaluation of a low bicarbonate level (Fig. 11–4). A low bicarbonate level may be a consequence of respiratory alkalosis with renal compensation. The pH determination will confirm if this is the case or if the patient indeed has acidosis.

Determination of Anion Gap. Once acidosis is confirmed, determination of the AG becomes the next issue.

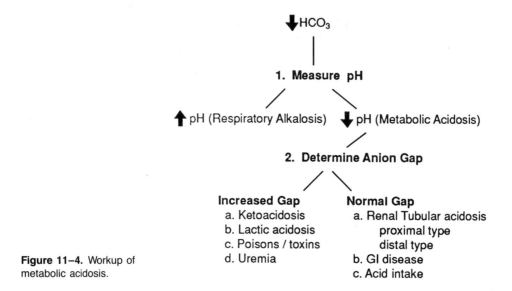

Figure 11–4. Workup of metabolic acidosis.

Clinical and Laboratory Assessment. Specific clinical and laboratory features can be used (Table 11–5) to ascertain which of the different causes of high or normal AG acidosis has developed.

Treatment

Seriousness. The first decision in determining the treatment of any acid-base disorder is to decide how harmful the abnormality in pH is to the patient. **Mild transient disorders usually have no adverse effects and do not require correction. Severe abnormalities, on the other hand, may be life-threatening and demand immediate treatment.**

Correcting the Disorder

Correct the Primary Cause. The second step in treatment is to decide whether the underlying disease responsible for the acid-base disorder can be corrected. If so, **the abnormality may be reversible without specific acid-base treatment.** For example, many cases of diabetic acidosis can be treated with insulin and appropriate intravenous fluids without supplemental bicarbonate.

Approach to Therapy. When specific therapy of acute metabolic acidosis is required, complete correction of the abnormality is not necessary. As in the treatment of other fluid and electrolyte disorders, **the goal is to correct the abnormality to a sufficient extent to eliminate its harmful effects on the patient,** an objective that usually can be achieved by **correction of the blood pH to about 7.2.** The severity of the disturbance determines the rate at which reversal of the

TABLE 11–5. EVALUATION OF METABOLIC ACIDOSIS

	History	Physical	Laboratory
Normal anion gap			
Excess acid intake	Parenteral nutrition or acidification treatment	—	—
Bicarbonate loss			
GI tract	Diarrhea, fistula	ECV depletion possible	
Kidney	Family history	—	Glycosuria common
Distal renal tubular acidosis	Renal stones History of diabetes	—	High urine pH (>5.6), high or low serum K+ with inappropriate urine K+
Increased anion gap			
Ketoacidosis	Diabetes Alcohol use	Odor of ketones Odor of alcohol	Hyperglycemia Increased blood alcohol
Lactic acidosis	Severely ill, CPR,[a] shock	Shock, sepsis, cardiac arrest	Increased blood lactate level
Poisons	Overdose, abnormal intake	Possible coma	Serum salicylate, urine oxalate crystals
Renal failure	—	Odor (urine)	Increased BUN and creatinine

[a]CPR, cardiopulmonary resuscitation.

abnormality should be attempted. As improvement occurs, the rate of alkali administration can be correspondingly tapered.

Avoid Overcorrection. A compelling reason for avoiding too rapid correction of a metabolic acid-base disorder is related to the effect of such a correction on spinal fluid pH. The **spinal fluid bicarbonate changes slowly in response to changes in plasma bicarbonate.** For example, if a patient with stable metabolic acidosis (low plasma bicarbonate and PCO_2) is treated rapidly with bicarbonate, the plasma concentration will return toward normal, the plasma pH will rise, and the plasma PCO_2 will quickly return toward normal also. In the spinal fluid, the PCO_2 rises toward normal because of rapid diffusion of CO_2 across the blood–brain barrier. However, bicarbonate in the CSF remains quite low. The result is a return of blood pH to normal but an accentuation of the acidosis in the spinal fluid. This situation may produce a worsening of the clinical picture, with development of coma and other neurologic signs.

Estimation of Acidosis. Only a rough estimate of the magnitude of the bicarbonate deficit in metabolic acidosis need be made, and it is of limited value to try to quantitate the amount of alkali that must be added to body fluids to correct the acidosis. There are two reasons for this uncertainty. First, the buffer capacity of the body is not accurately known in an individual. Second, the rate of acid production varies widely in different situations leading to metabolic acidosis. For example, in methanol intoxication, rapid infusion of bicarbonate may be necessary just to keep up with the rate of formic acid production. In acute renal failure, on the other hand, acid production may be limited to a normal rate of around 50 mEq/day, and only small amounts of bicarbonate are required to maintain homeostasis. For these reasons, calculations of bicarbonate deficit are inherently inaccurate, and therapy based on such calculations usually results in undershooting or overshooting the normal acid-base state. A rough estimate of the bicarbonate deficit can be made by subtracting the patient's measured bicarbonate from normal and multiplying this number by one-half the total body water. To repeat, **it is undesirable to attempt rapid correction of most cases of metabolic acidosis.**

Initiation of Therapy. Mild or chronic acidosis may be treated with oral bicarbonate. More severe cases should be given intravenous sodium bicarbonate. **In general, 50 mEq of bicarbonate (the amount in one ampule) will increase the serum bicarbonate by about 1 mEq in a 70 kg patient. However, since acid production may continue, it is wisest to give a dose and repeat blood gas determinations and decide on further doses according to the patient's response.**

METABOLIC ALKALOSIS

Causes

Sustained alkalosis usually results from excessive HCl loss from the stomach in the patient who is vomiting or from the urinary tract in a patient receiving diuretics (Table 11–6). Primary or secondary hyperaldosteronism will also enhance renal acid loss. Less frequently, excessive alkali intake or severe potassium depletion may be implicated. Usually, severe potassium depletion accompanies both extracellular volume (ECV) and HCl depletion, so the alkalosis is often of multifactorial origin.

TABLE 11–6. CAUSES OF METABOLIC ALKALOSIS

I. HCl loss
   A. Gastrointestinal (vomiting)
   B. Increased urine acidification
      1. Diuretics
      2. Aldosterone excess
      3. Bartter's syndrome
II. Excess alkali intake
   A. Alkali abuse (bicarbonate of soda self-administration)
   B. Treatment of acidosis
III. Severe potassium depletion

Figure 11–5 shows the primary factors leading to alkalosis with either diuretic use or vomiting. In both of these situations, chloride is lost in relatively higher proportions than it is present in the ECF. For instance, whereas chloride makes up about 70% of the anions in the ECF, it may comprise more than 90% of the anions lost in vomit or urine. The renal tubule is then forced to reabsorb or generate additional bicarbonate to maintain electrical neutrality.

In addition to volume and chloride depletion, which enhance proximal tubular bicarbonate reabsorption, there is HCl and KCl loss. Acid loss directly leads to alkalosis, whereas potassium depletion enhances hydrogen ion entry into cells, which, of course, contributes to ECF alkalosis.

In Figure 11–6, indirect effects of these primary disorders are depicted. These indirect effects make substantial contributions to causing or sustaining an alkalosis. Potassium depletion causes the shift of hydrogen ion into cells. Not only does this contribute to the alkalosis directly, but it also results in the tubular cells secreting acid, further worsening the alkalosis.

The ECV depletion also has indirect effects mediated through aldosterone. First, aldosterone enhances Na^+ reabsorption. Both K^+ and H^+ are exchanged for

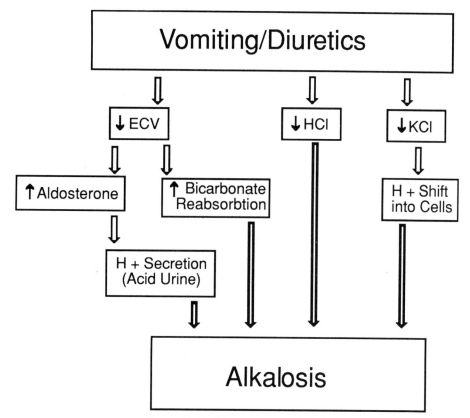

Figure 11–5. Primary causes of alkalosis.

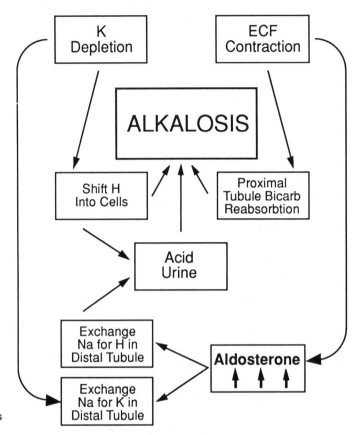

Figure 11–6. Secondary causes of alkalosis.

the reabsorbed Na$^+$, worsening the K$^+$ depletion and further enhancing renal acid loss, respectively.

Diagnosis and Workup

Evaluation of Bicarbonate Level. **There are no specific signs or symptoms.** As with most fluid disorders, the clinical history or setting may suggest that metabolic alkalosis is present. The serum bicarbonate level usually is the first clue to the presence of alkalosis. Again, as in metabolic acidosis, the **pH must be measured** to determine whether the excess bicarbonate is associated with metabolic alkalosis or is merely a compensatory response to a respiratory disturbance. Knowing the **patient's history** may obviate this. For instance, severe obstructive lung disease suggests a diagnosis of respiratory acidosis, whereas a history of vomiting or diuretic use suggests metabolic alkalosis. The urine pH is usually less than 7. This **paradoxical aciduria** (i.e., an acid urine in the face of ECF alkalosis) reflects the increased bicarbonate reabsorption and concomitant generation that must occur if alkalosis is to be sustained.

Extracellular Volume Status. Once metabolic alkalosis is confirmed, if the cause is not clear, the first thing to assess is the ECV status. A history of saline loss, evidence on examination, or a low urine sodium (< 30 mEq/day) all support ECV depletion. This should prompt evaluation of the mechanism of loss (usually vomiting or diuretic use or abuse).

One piece of laboratory data may be confusing in the patient who abuses diuretics. If someone has taken a diuretic recently, the urine sodium will be high. This would be paradoxical in a patient who otherwise appeared to be ECV depleted. After a few hours, when the diuretic is metabolized, the urine sodium will drop substantially and add supportive evidence to the clinical picture of ECV depletion.

If ECV depletion is not present, several relatively rare causes of alkalosis (Fig. 11–7) must be considered. For all of these, except Bartter's syndrome, a diagnosis usually can be made easily. Bartter's syndrome involves a specific tubular defect (in effect, renal tubular alkalosis), which is very difficult to confirm.

Potassium Depletion. Severe potassium depletion is an **unusual** cause of metabolic alkalosis that may be associated with either euvolemia or hypovolemia. It often is recognized when **correction of ECV depletion does not result in correction of the alkalosis.**

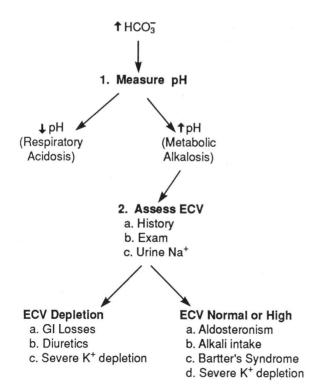

Figure 11–7. Workup of metabolic alkalosis.

Treatment

Mild to moderate alkalosis (blood pH < 7.55) rarely requires specific therapy.
When hypoxia also exists, it may be more urgent to correct the alkalosis to
decrease oxygen-hemoglobin affinity and improve tissue oxygenation. When ECF
and chloride deficiency are the cause of the alkalosis, the urinary chloride concentration is typically less than 10 mEq/L, and the disorder is responsive to volume
repletion with isosmolar sodium chloride. Rarely, severe gastric losses of hydrochloric acid may require intravenous therapy with ammonium chloride or even
dilute (0.1 to 0.2 mol/L) hydrochloric acid. Initial dosage should be based on
correction of the ECF bicarbonate excess, with additional doses dependent on
response (similar to metabolic acidosis, a rough estimate of bicarbonate excess can
be made by determining the difference between the patient's value and normal
value and multiplying that difference by one-half the total body water). However,
ammonium toxicity and phlebitis from hydrochloric acid limit the usefulness of
these agents. It is much more practical to prevent severe metabolic alkalosis from
gastric loss of hydrochloric acid by treatment with cimetidine, a histamine H_2-
receptor antagonist.

In the alkalosis associated with aldosteronism or severe potassium depletion,
ECF and chloride are not deficient, and the urinary chloride concentration reflects
dietary intake and typically exceeds 20 mEq/L. Alkalosis in such patients is chloride resistant and does not respond to sodium chloride. The alkalosis is correctable
with vigorous potassium therapy or, in the case of aldosteronism, correction of the
adrenal disorder or blockade with an aldosterone inhibitor.

RESPIRATORY DISORDERS

Respiratory Acidosis

Causes. This disorder results from **hypoventilation.** Because the production of
CO_2 is so high and chemical buffering is limited, **acute respiratory failure is
associated with severe acidosis and little increase in the plasma bicarbonate
concentration. However, chronic hypercapnia (high PCO_2) causes increased renal
generation of new bicarbonate at a rate of about 3 mEq/L for each 10 mm Hg
increment in the PCO_2 over the next several days.** This tends to ameliorate the
respiratory acidosis. The major causes of respiratory acidosis are noted in Table
11–7.

Clinical Findings. Clinical features are those accompanying **acute or chronic respiratory failure.** Hypoxia (low PO_2) frequently is associated and may be clinically
more important than the hypercapnia (high PCO_2). The diagnosis is established by
an elevated PCO_2. The degree of pH depression or plasma bicarbonate elevation
depends on whether the condition is acute or chronic (Fig. 11–2).

TABLE 11–7. CAUSES OF RESPIRATORY ACIDOSIS

I. Depression of respiratory center
   A. Strokes
   B. Tumors
   C. Encephalitis
   D. Drugs: Narcotics, sedatives, tranquilizers
II. Limitation of chest wall movement
   A. Neuromuscular disorders: myasthenia gravis, Guillain-Barré syndrome, tetanus
   B. Trauma and surgery
   C. Fixation of ribs
III. Pulmonary disease
   A. Chronic bronchitis
   B. Chronic emphysema
   C. Asthma
   D. Pneumonia

Treatment. **Improved ventilation is the mainstay of therapy.** This may require antibiotics, bronchodilators, or even mechanical ventilatory assistance.

Respiratory Alkalosis

Causes. Acute **hypocapnia (low PCO_2)** causes a release of intracellular hydrogen ion from tissue buffers. This tends to minimize the alkalosis and causes a small reduction in plasma bicarbonate concentration. Chronic hypocapnia stimulates renal adaptation with reduced bicarbonate generation, thus lowering the plasma bicarbonate concentration. **This disorder results from hyperventilation** due to a variety of causes, as shown in Table 11–8.

TABLE 11–8. CAUSES OF RESPIRATORY ALKALOSIS

I. Direct stimulation of respiratory center
   A. Psychogenic
   B. CNS disease: Stroke, encephalitis
   C. Sepsis (gram-negative, particularly)
   D. Hypermetabolic state: Fever, thyrotoxicosis, delirium tremens
   E. Exercise
   F. Liver failure
   G. Drugs: Salicylates, ammonia, progesterone
II. Reflex (hypoxemia) stimulation of respiratory center
   A. Pneumonia
   B. Pulmonary edema
   C. Pulmonary fibrosis
   D. Asthma
   E. Cyanotic heart disease
III. Excessive mechanical ventilation

Clinical Findings. Symptoms of **irritability, light-headedness, paresthesia, tetany, and even syncope** may occur with acute respiratory alkalosis. **Hyperventilation may not be clinically apparent.** The laboratory finding of a low PCO_2 associated with reduction of plasma bicarbonate and increased pH makes the diagnosis.

Treatment. Successful treatment must be directed toward the precipitating cause. Symptoms associated with acute hyperventilation may be relieved by rebreathing into a paper bag. Occasionally, sedation or a CO_2 rebreathing apparatus may be used for chronic hypocapnia.

MIXED DISORDERS

In acutely ill patients, two acid-base problems often coexist. It may be difficult to sort out the disorders; the blood gases, AG, and clinical setting are all important indices. Some of the more common mixed disorders are listed in Table 11–9.

Many physicians find the nomogram (Fig. 11–2) useful in helping to determine a patient's acid-base condition. The pH, PCO_2, and HCO_3^- are simply plot-

TABLE 11–9. COMMON MIXED ACID-BASE DISORDERS

Disorder	Clinical Setting	pH	Pco₂	HCO₃⁻	Anion Gap
Respiratory acidosis and metabolic alkalosis	COPD and vomiting or diuretics	Normal to high	High	High	Normal
Respiratory acidosis and metabolic acidosis	Cardiac arrest; sepsis, pneumonia and lactic acid; drug overdose with shock and hypoventilation	Very low	High	Low	High
	COPD and any metabolic acidosis	Low	High	Low	Varies
Respiratory alkalosis and metabolic acidosis	Aspirin toxicity; early sepsis: hyperventilation and lactic acid	Normalᵃ	Low	Low	High
Respiratory alkalosis and metabolic alkalosis	GI loss and mechanical ventilation	High	Low	High	Normal
Metabolic acidosis and metabolic alkalosis	Diarrhea and vomiting; vomiting or diuretics and any metabolic acidosis	Normalᵃ Normalᵃ	Normal Normal	Normal Normal	Normal Varies
Respiratory alkalosis and metabolic acidosis and metabolic alkalosis (the triple ripple)	Alcoholic with cirrhosis (hyperventilation) and vomiting and alcoholic ketoacidosis	Normalᵃ to slightly high	Low	Normal to high	High

ᵃIf one disorder is more severe, the numbers will more closely resemble that disorder.

ted on the graph. The use of this nomogram is not a panacea for diagnosing all acid-base disorders, nor does it obviate the need for clinical evaluation.

STUDY CASES

Case 1

History. This 48-year-old man has a long history of peptic ulcer and recently began to vomit frequently. X-ray studies demonstrated pyloric obstruction.

Physical Examination. Weight 76 kg (usual 74 kg), temperature 37°C, respirations 14, pulse 84, blood pressure 140/80 (supine) and 135/85 (sitting). No remarkable findings were noted on examination.

Laboratory Data. Hct 38%, serum sodium 130, potassium 2.8, chloride 82, HCO_3^- 38, glucose 82, urea nitrogen 12, creatinine 1.1 mg/dL. Urinalysis unremarkable. Arterial blood: pH 7.51, PCO_2 55, PO_2 85. Fluid balance for the past 24 hours is recorded.

	Input		Output		
Volume	4000	mL	2600	mL	Urine
Na+	300	mEq	1000	ml	S & I
K+	80	mEq	1800	mL	GI
Cl/HCO3	380	mEq	5400	mL	Total

1. What fluid and electrolyte problems are present?
2. Explain the pathogenesis of the arterial blood abnormalities.
3. What is the significance, if any, of the weight change?
4. Estimate the urine electrolytes.
5. Plan treatment for the next 24 hours on the blank flow sheet below and on next page.

BASIC ALLOWANCE						
	Volume	Na+	K+	H+	Cl-	HCO3-
Urine						
S + I						
GI						
TOTAL:						

DIAGNOSES:
1. ECV (Saline)
2. Water
3. Acid/Base
4. Potassium

Corrections	Volume	Na+	K+	H+	Cl-	HCO3-
Saline +/-			▓▓▓▓	▓▓▓▓		▓▓▓▓
Water +/-		▓▓▓▓	▓▓▓▓	▓▓▓▓	▓▓▓▓	▓▓▓▓
Acid/Base +/-						
Potassium +/-	▓▓▓▓	▓▓▓▓				
SUM: Basics + Corrections						

Case 2

History. A 39-year-old woman with a 16-year history of diabetes mellitus was admitted because of persistent vomiting. She had been well and was without known complications of diabetes. Four days previously, she developed a flu-like syndrome and had been vomiting since. Her usual insulin dose was 45 to 50 units of Lente insulin daily, but she had decreased her dose to 20 units daily when she was unable to eat.

Physical Examination. She was lethargic and somnolent but responsive to questions. Blood pressure 188/70 lying, 110/40 sitting. Respirations were deep and regular at 24/minute. Temperature 37°C. Weight 56 kg (usual 61 kg). An odor of acetone was noted on her breath. Neck veins were flat in the supine position. The skin turgor was poor. The abdomen was distended and tympanitic, with hypoactive bowel sounds. A supine abdominal roentgenogram showed distended bowel loops with fluid levels.

Laboratory Data. Hct 45%, WBC 34,000, serum sodium 134, potassium 6.4, chloride 100, bicarbonate 9 mEq/L, glucose 1100, urea nitrogen 60, creatinine 3 mg/dL. Serum amylase 10 U/mL. Urinalysis: Sp. gr. 1.040, pH 6, protein 300 mg/dL, glucose 4+, ketones 4+; sediment showed pyuria, renal tubular cells with fat, and many granular casts. Arterial blood: pH 7.18, P_{CO_2} 25. The serum acetone was weakly positive in a 1:16 dilution.

6. What fluid and electrolyte problems are present?

7. How does the finding of azotemia influence initial therapy?

A nasogastric tube was inserted. During the next 4 hours, the patient received crystalline insulin intravenously at a rate of 10 units/hour and the fluid therapy noted below. She improved markedly. Skin turgor was better, neck veins became visible while lying, and the postural blood pressure fall lessened. The patient continued to have over 2% (4+) glucosuria. Actual intake and output data were as follows.

Intake			Output		
Volume	3000	mL	200	mL	Urine
Na+	432	mEq	250	mL	S+I (est.)
K+	0		500	mL	GI
Cl-	388	mEq	950	mL	Total
HCO3-	44	mEq			

BASIC ALLOWANCE						
	Volume	Na+	K+	H+	Cl-	HCO3-
Urine				▨		▨
S + I		▨	▨	▨	▨	▨
GI						
TOTAL:						

DIAGNOSES:
1. ECV (Saline)
2. Water
3. Acid/Base
4. Potassium

Corrections	Volume	Na+	K+	H+	Cl-	HCO3-
Saline +/-			▨	▨		▨
Water +/-		▨	▨	▨	▨	▨
Acid/Base +/-						
Potassium +/-	▨					
SUM: Basics + Corrections						

At 4:00 PM, laboratory results were as follows: blood glucose 600 mg/dL, serum sodium 149, potassium 3.2, chloride 115, bicarbonate 17 mEq/L, urea nitrogen 59, creatinine 2.9 mg/dL.

8. Comment on the therapy given and the current fluid and electrolyte status.

9. Plan therapy for the next *4 hours* using the blank worksheet.

Case 3

History. A 35-year-old man was brought to the emergency room by ambulance. He had been found in a stuporous state by friends at a downtown hotel. There was little history available except that he was thought to have been on an alcoholic binge recently. Past medical records contained a history of peptic ulcer disease and frequent alcoholic binges.

Physical Examination. Rectal temperature 39°C, respirations 18, pulse 150, blood pressure 95/60 (supine) and unmeasurable while sitting. He was obtunded but arousable. Skin turgor was poor, and neck veins were not visible in the lying position. The left chest was dull, with rales posteriorly. A chest x-ray film showed an infiltrate in the left lower lobe. Bowel sounds were hypoactive, and tenderness was noted in the epigastrium. The rectal examination was negative except for hematochezia (1+ guaiac reaction). No edema was seen.

Laboratory Data. Hct 40%, WBC 6000 with 70% polys, serum sodium 125, potassium 3.0, chloride 75, bicarbonate 25 mEq/L, glucose 200, urea nitrogen 10, creatinine 1.8 mg/dL. Arterial blood: pH 7.41, P_{CO_2} 40. Urinalysis: pH 6.5, Sp. gr. 1.012, protein 30 mg/dL, negative for glucose, ketones, and blood; sediment contained a few granular casts.

10. What fluid and electrolyte problems are present? Discuss the possible etiology of each.

Course. Several hours after infusion of isotonic sodium chloride, the patient's mentation improved, and the lying blood pressure was 115/75 without a postural fall. Laboratory values were Hct 35%, serum sodium 127, potassium 2.5, chloride 82, bicarbonate 35 mEq/L, glucose 150, urea nitrogen 8, creatinine 1.5. Arterial blood: pH 7.56, P_{CO_2} 41, P_{O_2} 60.

11. What is the current fluid and electrolyte status? What is the probable reason for these changes?
12. Plan therapy on the blank worksheet.

BASIC ALLOWANCE	Volume	Na+	K+	H+	Cl-	HCO3-
Urine						
S + I						
GI						
TOTAL:						

DIAGNOSES:
1. ECV (Saline)
2. Water
3. Acid/Base
4. Potassium

Corrections	Volume	Na+	K+	H+	Cl-	HCO3-
Saline +/-						
Water +/-						
Acid/Base +/-						
Potassium +/-						
SUM: Basics + Corrections						

ACID-BASE PUZZLERS

Directions. The goal of this is to match three sets of data: (1) the patient profile (1,2,3. . . 7), (2) the acid-base disorder (A, B. . . F), and (3) the single most appropriate set of laboratory data (a, b. . . h). Since more than one type of acid-base disorder may be present, the letters A through F may be used more than once and in any combination you think is most likely. Letters are not to be used for adaptive or compensatory changes.

Patient Profile

1. A 42-year-old comatose, hyperventilating woman with diabetes mellitus
2. A 62-year-old man with chronic renal failure and severe pneumococcal pneumonia
3. A 55-year-old woman with glaucoma who is receiving acetazolamide (Diamox)
4. A 16-year-old boy who had taken an overdose of sedative and was brought to the emergency room with shallow respiration
5. A 48-year-old woman with severe emphysema
6. A 46-year-old woman who ingested a full bottle of aspirin tablets
7. A 35-year-old man who is vomiting due to a gastric outlet obstruction

Acid-Base Disorder

A. Metabolic acidosis
B. Metabolic alkalosis
C. Chronic respiratory acidosis
D. Acute respiratory acidosis
E. Chronic respiratory alkalosis
F. Acute respiratory alkalosis

Laboratory Data

	Na	K	Cl	HCO_3	Anion Gap	pH	PCO_2	PO_2
a.	128	3.7	101	16	11	7.46	25	85
b.	138	3.8	101	7	30	7.20	20	92
c.	141	3.4	115	16	10	7.35	31	88
d.	135	3.1	95	32	8	7.48	46	70
e.	137	5.1	105	14	18	7.15	40	55
f.	139	3.8	101	26	12	7.32	55	62
g.	137	4.1	90	36	11	7.34	71	71
h.	146	3.5	106	20	20	7.55	25	96

Serum columns: Na, K, Cl, HCO_3. Arterial columns: pH, PCO_2, PO_2.

ANSWERS TO STUDY CASES

Case 1

1. What fluid and electrolyte problems are present?

ECF. No objective evidence of depletion noted despite history of vomiting.

Water. Serum sodium concentration is low. In view of normal serum glucose, the hyponatremia reflects cellular swelling and a state of relative water excess of about 3L (see Chapter 10 for calculations). Probably ADH is being secreted in response to ECV depletion which is not sufficient to detect clinically.

Acid-base. The history of gastric fluid loss plus an elevated serum bicarbonate and arterial pH are all compatible with metabolic alkalosis. The P_{CO_2} is increased because of adaptive hypoventilation. The anion gap is normal. There is, thus, no evidence of other significant acid-base disorders. The bicarbonate excess approximately is

$$\text{(Patient bicarbonate} - \text{normal bicarbonate) (TBW/2)} = (38 - 25) (42/2)$$
$$= 13 \times 21 = 273 \text{ mEq}$$

Potassium. The serum level is low and is corrected partially by adjustments for the arterial pH. However, the low corrected value reflects a total body depletion of about 10% or 300 mEq.

2. Explain the pathogenesis of the arterial blood abnormalities.

The problem is initiated by loss of hydrochloric acid in gastric fluid. The loss of hydrion causes an alkalosis, and the chloride depletion prevents the kidney from excreting bicarbonate. The high P_{CO_2} is caused by the alkalosis depressing the respiratory center. Despite hypoventilation, however, oxygen exchange is adequate. Although orthostatic blood pressure changes are not present, the body probably is responding to some degree of ECV depletion by releasing aldosterone.

3. What is the significance, if any, of the weight change?

The weight gain appears to be explained by a small loss of saline-containing fluid from vomiting plus retention of about 3L of solute-free water.

4. Estimate the urine electrolytes.

Because of sub-clinical hypovolemia with secondary aldosteronism, urine sodium would be low and potassium would be moderately high.

5. Plan treatment for the next 24 hours.

The problems noted can be corrected by administration of sodium and potassium chloride. See fluid balance worksheet 11–1 for a possible approach. Note

BASIC ALLOWANCE

	Volume	Na+	K+	H+	Cl-	HCO3-
Urine	1500	50	40		90	
S + I	1000					
GI	1800	180	18		198	
TOTAL:	4300	230	58		288	

DIAGNOSES:
1. ECV (Saline) NORMAL
2. Water EXCESS
3. Acid/Base METABOLIC ALKALOSIS
4. Potassium DEPLETION

Corrections	Volume	Na+	K+	H+	Cl-	HCO3-
Saline +/-						
Water +/-	-1000					
Acid/Base +/-	+2000	+300			+300	
Potassium +/-			+100		+100	
SUM: Basics + Corrections	5300	530	158		688	

Worksheet 11–1. Fluid balance worksheet, Case 1, answers.

that in this case, saline is used to provide chloride to correct alkalosis and not for volume depletion. As noted previously, there is no doubt a small amount of subclinical volume depletion that also will be corrected. This type of problem may be ameliorated in part also by the use of cimetidine, an H_2 antagonist. Cimetidine reduces hydrochloric acid production and, hence, the loss of acid that occurs when nasogastric suction is used as a part of medical therapy for pyloric obstruction.

Case 2

6. What fluid and electrolyte problems are present?

ECF. Physical findings of postural hypotension, flat neck veins, and poor skin turgor are compatible with ECF depletion. The physical findings are compatible with the history of gastrointestinal fluid loss by vomiting and uncontrolled diabetes mellitus. The elevated serum urea nitrogen and creatinine suggest that the ECF deficit is causing prerenal azotemia, but she may also have renal failure from diabetic nephropathy.

Water. A deficit is present. Serum sodium is low normal at 134 mEq/L. However, when corrected for hyperglycemia

$$\frac{(Glucose)\,(2)}{100} = 22$$

the corrected serum sodium is 156 mEq/L. She is effectively hypernatremic, indicating a water deficit. The osmotic diuresis from glucosuria results in loss of urinary water, with a urine sodium concentration of 100 mEq/L or less. This is the reason for hypernatremia.

Acid-Base. The patient has severe metabolic acidosis (arterial pH 7.18) caused by ketoacidosis from uncontrolled diabetes mellitus. The anion gap is elevated to 25, which is compatible with diabetic ketoacidosis and confirmed by a positive serum acetone out to a 1:16 dilution. Her deep, regular breathing is typical of respiratory adaptation for metabolic acidosis when pulmonary function is normal. Her bicarbonate deficit is 288 mEq.

Potassium. The hyperkalemia of 6.4 mEq/L is caused by the acidosis. If it is corrected for the pH of 7.18, the serum potassium is in the normal range. Thus, no true potassium excess is present.

Hyperglycemia and renal function. As long as GFR is normal, the plasma glucose does not exceed 700 to 800 mg/dL. At this plasma level, the urinary glucose excreted plus that metabolized is equal to the rate of production. However, if the GFR falls from functional or intrinsic renal disease, higher levels of hyperglycemia are typical when severe uncontrolled diabetes mellitus occurs. In this patient, the impaired renal function (serum creatinine of 3 mg/dL) probably reflects both prerenal azotemia from the ECF depletion and diabetic nephropathy (proteinuria, oval fat bodies, granular casts). The pyuria not only may be caused by the diabetic nephropathy but also could reflect a urinary tract infection.

7. How does the finding of azotemia influence initial therapy?

In the presence of renal failure, unknown urine output, and hyperkalemia, parenteral potassium is not given. Such therapy is started after the serum potassium is normal (corrected for arterial pH) and the urinary output is reasonable.

8. Comment on the therapy given and the current fluid and electrolyte status.

ECF. The deficit previously noted (caused in part by water depletion) has been largely corrected by the isotonic saline given.

Water. Unfortunately, no solute-free water was given, and the deficit previously noted (about 4 L) is still present.

Acid-base. A metabolic acidosis is still present but is slowly improving with current insulin therapy. Parenteral bicarbonate is no longer needed.

Potassium. The fall in the serum level to a hypokalemic value reflects mainly cellular uptake. It now appears safe and necessary to give parenteral potassium in view of body depletion.

BASIC ALLOWANCE	Volume	Na+	K+	H+	Cl-	HCO3-
Urine	250	10	8	▓▓▓	18	▓▓▓
S + I	200	▓▓▓	▓▓▓		▓▓▓	▓▓▓
GI	500	50	5		55	
TOTAL:	950	60	13		73	

DIAGNOSES:
1. ECV (Saline) CORRECTED
2. Water DEPLETION
3. Acid/Base ACIDOSIS
4. Potassium DEPLETION

Corrections	Volume	Na+	K+	H+	Cl-	HCO3-
Saline +/-	+500	+75	▓▓▓	▓▓▓	+75	▓▓▓
Water +/-	+500	▓▓▓	▓▓▓	▓▓▓	▓▓▓	▓▓▓
Acid/Base +/-						
Potassium +/-	▓▓▓	▓▓▓	+80		+80	
SUM: Basics + Corrections	1950	175	93		153	

Worksheet 11–2. Fluid balance worksheet, Case 2, answers.

9. Plan therapy for the next 4 hours.

The ECF is still depleted and needs further expansion. Hyposmolar solutions also are needed to correct water depletion. The metabolic acidosis has decreased and will be corrected if insulin therapy is continued and ketones are metabolized. A clear-cut potassium depletion is now evident and requires treatment. A possible plan is shown in the fluid balance worksheet 11–2.

Case 3

10. What fluid and electrolyte problems are present? Discuss the possible etiology of each.

ECF. The supine and postural hypotension, flat neck veins, and poor skin turgor are consistent with a reduced ECF, even in the absence of a history of fluid loss. Thus, mild azotemia (serum creatinine 1.8 mg/dL) may be due to prerenal factors, since the urinalysis is not suggestive of primary renal disease. The serum urea nitrogen/creatinine ratio is low and suggests that urea production has been suppressed by the ingestion of nonprotein calories or liver disease.

The lack of elevation of the hematocrit is suggestive of an underlying anemia, which could be due to folate deficiency as commonly seen in the alcoholic and red cell loss from gastrointestinal bleeding. Although speculative, the most likely cause of the ECF deficit is a loss from the gastrointestinal tract, most likely vomiting.

Water. Hyponatremia is present, but the serum glucose is elevated. However, correction for the elevated glucose (as explained in the text and the previous case) would only raise the serum sodium by 3 mEq. Thus, there is evidence of relative water excess and cell swelling. This finding often is seen in patients who have been vomiting and have become ECF depleted. It is probably related to a release of ADH and an intrinsic change in salt and water handling by the kidney, leading to an inability to excrete a dilute urine with customary water ingestion.

Acid-base. On the surface, this patient appears to be normal, but the elevated anion gap (25 mEq/L) reveals an underlying metabolic acidosis. The only way in which a metabolic acidosis could be present and the arterial pH and PCO_2 remain normal is to have an equal amount of metabolic alkalosis. The reason for the metabolic acidosis is unclear, but in the absence of ketoacidosis, significant azotemia, or a history of salicylate or methanol ingestion, it is most likely that this represents some other organic acidosis. The etiology for metabolic alkalosis is also unknown, but it is most likely caused by a loss of hydrochloric acid from vomiting.

Potassium. The serum potassium is low and, at an arterial pH of 7.4, is compatible with a 10% body depletion. The loss is undoubtedly due to poor intake in the presence of gastrointestinal and renal losses.

11. What is the current fluid and electrolyte status? What is the probable reason for these changes?

ECF. ECF appears normal now after adequate expansion with isotonic sodium chloride.

Water. The patient is still hyponatremic from relative water excess. This should improve with water restriction and improving renal function now that ECF repair has occurred.

Acid-base. The metabolic acidosis is now gone (anion gap equals 10). The rapidity of its disappearance suggests an organic acid (e.g., acetate, lactate, beta-hydroxybutyrate) that was metabolized after tissue circulation improved. The underlying metabolic alkalosis, probably related to vomiting, is now evident and will require chloride repletion.

Potassium. Although the serum concentration is lower, this is caused by the elevation of arterial pH. The degree of depletion is substantially unchanged.

BASIC ALLOWANCE							
	Volume	Na+	K+	H+	Cl-	HCO3-
Urine	1500	50	40	▓▓▓▓▓	90	▓▓▓▓▓
S + I	1000	▓▓▓▓▓				
GI						
TOTAL:	2500	50	40		90	

DIAGNOSES:
1. ECV (Saline) CORRECTED
2. Water EXCESS
3. Acid/Base METABOLIC ALKALOSIS
4. Potassium DEPLETION

Corrections	Volume	Na+	K+	H+	Cl-	HCO3-
Saline +/-			▓▓▓▓▓			▓▓▓▓▓
Water +/-	-1000	▓▓▓▓▓	▓▓▓▓▓	▓▓▓▓▓	▓▓▓▓▓	▓▓▓▓▓
Acid/Base +/-		+150			+150	
Potassium +/-	▓▓▓▓▓		+20		+20	
SUM: Basics + Corrections	1500	200	60		260	

Worksheet 11-3. Fluid balance worksheet, Case 3, answers.

12. Plan therapy.

A possible treatment plan is shown on fluid balance worksheet 11-3. It is based on sufficient water restriction to give only isotonic saline correction plus potassium chloride supplementation.

ANSWERS TO ACID-BASE PUZZLERS

Patient	Acid-Base Disorder	Laboratory Data
1	A	b
2	A + D (Lack of respiratory compensation)	e
3	A	c
4	D	f
5	C	g
6	A + F	h
7	B	d

Comment on Acid-Base Puzzlers: The point of this exercise is to attempt to correlate the laboratory and clinical information. Close attention to the acid-base nomogram (Fig. 11-2) should be helpful.

Case Analysis

1. This woman in coma who is hyperventilating and has known diabetes mellitus ought to have ketoacidosis, a metabolic acidosis with a large anion gap. With hyperventilation, one would expect a low P_{CO_2}. An alternative possibility would be a stroke causing both hyperventilation and coma. In this case, she would have respiratory alkalosis and a normal anion gap, quite a different picture.

2. In this setting, one would expect both an increased anion gap metabolic acidosis (due to renal failure) and a respiratory acidosis (due to respiratory failure). This combined disorder results in the most severe acidosis in the possibilities given. A P_{CO_2} of 40 (laboratory data e) does not seem to represent much pulmonary disease. However, if one looks at Figure 11–2, it is apparent that a P_{CO_2} between 20 and 30 would be the expected respiratory compensation for this low a bicarbonate level. The pneumonia prevents adequate compensation.

3. Diamox is an older therapy for glaucoma. It is a carbonic anhydrase inhibitor. A complication of its use is impaired renal bicarbonate reabsorption. With renal bicarbonate wasting (proximal renal tubular acidosis), a nonanion gap metabolic acidosis occurs. Respiratory compensation should result in a lowered P_{CO_2}.

4. Assuming from the information that the only problem is the suppressed breathing, an acute respiratory acidosis is likely. Because renal compensation is sluggish, a near normal bicarbonate would probably be present with an elevated P_{CO_2} and no anion gap. Another alternative would be if the patient had taken a large enough dose to cause shock. In this case, lactic acidosis could coexist as a result of poor tissue perfusion.

5. This patient should have chronic respiratory acidosis (low pH, high P_{CO_2}), and a high bicarbonate from the expected renal compensation, with no anion gap, of course.

6. Aspirin has a mixed effect. It is an acid with an unmeasured ion. Thus, one would expect an increased anion gap and a metabolic acidosis. Aspirin also is a respiratory stimulant and causes a respiratory alkalosis. The pH that occurs is quite variable from individual to individual. Often, the respiratory disorder predominates early, giving an alkalosis, and the metabolic disorder supervenes after several hours.

7. In this case, one would expect acid to be lost. Therefore, the bicarbonate would rise, as would the pH (metabolic alkalosis). A small rise in P_{CO_2} (Fig. 11–7 and Table 11–3) would also occur as breathing is suppressed a bit to compensate.

Obstructive Uropathy

INTRODUCTION

Urinary tract obstruction is a common problem in urology and an important cause of renal failure. Infection and stone formation are complications of obstruction and may lead to rapid renal deterioration. Because the adverse effects of obstruction may occur in patients of any age, diagnosis and relief of obstruction are problems concerning clinicians in all fields of medicine.

STUDY QUESTIONS

1. Define obstructive uropathy and explain the significance of this condition.
2. Classify the potential causes of obstructive uropathy.
3. Give two examples of each major cause of obstruction in Question 2.
4. Explain the effects of obstruction on the urinary tract.
5. Explain the nature and significance of postobstructive diuresis.

DEFINITION, CAUSES, AND CLASSIFICATION

Definition
Obstructive uropathy is the term used to describe the effects of blockage of the urinary stream on the structure and function of the urinary tract. This process may occur at any level of the urinary tract from the glomerulus, where urine is initially filtered, to the fossa navicularis, where urine leaves the penis in males, or to the distal urethra in females.

Causes
The causes of **obstructive uropathy may be classified as either anatomic or functional. Anatomic obstruction results from discrete mechanical lesions that block the flow of urine.** A stone lodged at the entry of the ureter into the bladder (the ureterovesical junction) is a good example of an anatomic obstruction. **Functional obstruction results from disturbance of the normal transport of the urine in the absence of an anatomic blockage.** For example, abnormal contraction of the bladder outlet may occur during voiding in patients with neurologic or psychologic disorders, leading to extremely high resistance to urine flow.

Classification
To help direct diagnostic evaluation and treatment it is useful to consider the causes of obstructive uropathy according to the following scheme.

    1. Anatomic problem?
        a. Congenital or acquired?
        b. Intrinsic or extrinsic?
    2. Functional problem?

Anatomic Causes. There are many anatomic causes of obstructive uropathy. Each of these conditions may be considered as either congenital or acquired and also as either intrinsic or extrinsic (Table 12–1).

Congenital Anomalies. Congenital anomalies affect the genitourinary tract more frequently than any other organ system and represent the most common cause of anatomic **obstruction in children.** The developing kidneys are especially susceptible to obstructive uropathy. Severe dilation of the renal pelvis and calyces, termed **hydronephrosis, is particularly damaging during the neonatal period** because the

TABLE 12–1. COMMON ANATOMIC CAUSES OF OBSTRUCTIVE UROPATHY

Level of Obstruction	Congenital		Acquired	
	Intrinsic	**Extrinsic**	**Intrinsic**	**Extrinsic**
Ureter	Ureteropelvic junction obstruction[a] Ureterovesical junction obstruction Ureterocele	Ureteropelvic junction obstruction[a] Retrocaval ureter	Stone[a] Inflammation Injury Papillary necrosis Tumor	Retroperitoneal fibrosis Aortic aneurism Pregnancy Uterine fibroid Injury Retroperitoneal tumor
Bladder neck	Ureterocele	Bowel abnormalities	Benign prostatic hypertrophy (BPH)[a] Prostate cancer[a] Bladder cancer Bladder stone	Cervical cancer Colon cancer Injury
Urethra	Posterior valves Phimosis Stricture Meatal stenosis		Stricture[a] Carcinoma of urethra Urethral stone Phimosis	Injury

[a]Most frequent causes.

Data from Wyker AW, Jr, Gillenwater JY: Method of Urology. *Baltimore: Williams and Wilkins; 1975.*

adverse effects of obstruction will have begun in utero, starting at the time of initial urine formation during the fourth month of development. Common sites of congenital obstruction are the origin of the ureter from the pelvis (**ureteropelvic junction obstruction**), the entry of the ureter into the bladder (**ureterovesical junction obstruction**), the posterior urethra (**posterior urethral valves**), and the urethral meatus (**meatal stenosis and phimosis**).

Acquired abnormalities. In **adults,** acquired lesions account for most mechanical obstructions to urinary flow. Common acquired causes of urinary tract obstruction include **stones, cancers** of the bladder or prostate, **benign prostatic hypertrophy (BPH),** and **urethral stricture.** Stones tend to cause symptoms when they become impacted at narrow points along the urinary conduit: the ureteropelvic junction, the level of the iliac vessels, the ureterovesical junction, and the bladder neck. Local extension of cancers of the bladder and prostate may cause obstruction of the ureteral orifices or bladder outlet. BPH may cause symptoms of urinary frequency and urgency. BPH also may present as urinary retention, in which the patient is acutely uncomfortable due to total inability to void (acute retention) or has sustained damage to his renal function (chronic retention). **Urethral strictures** are fibrotic scars of the urethra, resulting from infection or trauma, that may block urine flow and cause urinary retention.

Intrinsic Versus Extrinsic Problems. Anatomic causes of obstructive uropathy may be classified further as either intrinsic lesions or extrinsic lesions, based on their **origin either within or external to the urinary tract,** respectively. Each of the abnormalities discussed previously originated within the urinary system itself and, therefore, may be considered as intrinsic lesions. Disease processes in other organ systems also may lead to urinary tract obstruction. For example, the ureters often are obstructed in patients with inflammatory conditions, such as retroperitoneal fibrosis. Another example is ureteral compression at the level of the pelvic brim caused by metastatic nodes from prostate or cervical cancer. Because the primary pathology in these cases originates outside the urinary tract, such conditions are considered extrinsic causes of obstructive uropathy.

Functional Causes. Functional problems may cause obstructive uropathy in the **absence of anatomic obstruction** and, in extreme cases, may even result in secondary mechanical obstruction. To understand how functional abnormalities may cause obstructive uropathy, it is necessary to review the normal physiology of urinary transport and storage.

Normal Function of the Collecting and Voiding System

TRANSPORT OF URINE IN THE UPPER URINARY TRACT. The urinary collecting system begins at the renal papilla, which has an inner mucosal layer surrounded by a circular layer of smooth muscle. The smooth muscle layer contracts intermittently, propelling urine from the papilla into first the calyces then the renal pelvis. Periodic contractions of the renal pelvis cause boluses of urine to flow through the ureteropelvic junction into the ureter.

The normal pressure in the renal pelvis is less than 13 cm H_2O at the usual rates of urine flow but may increase to 20 cm H_2O during diuresis. Normally, the lower two thirds of the ureter are empty at rest, with intermittent distention as the urine bolus passes through. The intraureteric pressures may increase to 20 cm H_2O during passage of the urinary bolus (**peristaltic waves**), but closure of the ureter behind the bolus prevents transmission of the pressure wave to the renal pelvis. There is a valvelike mechanism at the ureteropelvic junction that allows urine to pass into the bladder but prevents reflux of urine from the bladder back into the ureter.

STORAGE AND TRANSPORT OF URINE IN THE LOWER URINARY TRACT. The **bladder serves as a reservoir** for storage of urine and should contract only at an appropriate time and place. Immediately after voiding, the bladder should be empty, with a pressure < 10 cm H_2O. Urine enters from the ureters, but there is little change in pressure and no contraction of the bladder musculature until the bladder is nearly full (normally around 400 to 600 mL). This **characteristic increase in capacity with minimal increase in pressure is called accommodation.** There is an increase in pressure near capacity as the elastic limit of the bladder is reached. The characteristics of the bladder during filling may be measured by obtaining a cystometrogram (Figure 12–1).

NORMAL CYSTOMETROGRAM

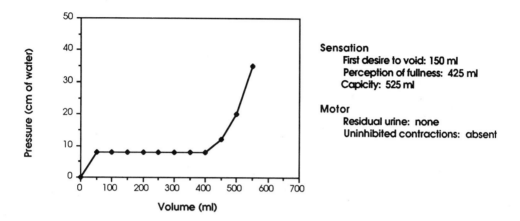

Figure 12–1. Cystometrogram in a patient with normal bladder function.

Continence means that urine is retained in the bladder until the patient desires to void. Continence depends on intact bladder function, that is, absence of involuntary contractions during filling plus the ability to initiate a sustained contraction, when desired, to achieve adequate voiding. In addition, continence depends on the resistance to drainage of urine provided by the urinary sphincters.

The **urinary sphincters are located at the bladder outlet and urethra.** Anatomically, the sphincters are ill defined, but functionally there appear to be three general mechanisms: (1) the bladder neck, (2) the intrinsic urethral mechanism, and (3) the extrinsic urethral mechanism. The bladder neck appears to be the primary sphincter. However, if the bladder neck is open (e.g., in a man who has had a prostatectomy), continence is maintained in the urethra. This distal sphincter has two elements, an intrinsic mechanism and an extrinsic mechanism. The intrinsic mechanism is composed of elastic tissue and smooth muscle at the level of the pelvic floor. The voluntary (striated) external sphincter is the second element of the distal continence mechanism. The external sphincter serves mainly to interrupt the urinary stream voluntarily and to maintain continence during sudden increases in intraabdominal pressure, for example, with coughing.

The **nervous control** of bladder filling and voiding is complex and under the control of the **S2–S4 reflex arcs.** During the filling phase, the bladder serves as a low pressure reservoir and does not exhibit involuntary contractions. The bladder sphincters maintain continence by exerting higher pressure than is present in the bladder itself. The initial event in voiding is voluntary relaxation of the pelvic floor and bladder neck. This reduces the resistance to urinary outflow. Coordinated contraction of the detrusor then opens the sphincters. Detrusor contraction continues until the bladder is empty. In summary, **control of lower urinary tract function depends on the integrated interplay of muscular and neurologic structures.**

Functional Obstruction of the Urinary Tract. Conceptually, there are three problems with urinary tract function that may lead to obstruction of the urinary stream: (1) abnormalities in transmission of the bolus of urine within the upper tract, (2) anatomic abnormalities inhibiting drainage of the ureters into the bladder, and (3) neurogenic abnormalities affecting the lower urinary tract.

ABNORMAL PERISTALSIS IN THE UPPER URINARY TRACT. Because generation of adequate peristalsis in the ureter is the chief mechanism for transmission of urine from the kidneys to the bladder, **any process that inhibits peristalsis may result in physiologic obstruction** of the urinary flow. Transmission of the peristaltic wave within the ureter depends on the ability of the ureter to glide within its adventitia. Immobilization of any portion of the ureter results in loss of this ability to move freely and may lead to obstruction. **Fibrosis** due to inflammation or prior surgery and **tumors** arising from other abdominal or retroperitoneal structures are examples of conditions that may cause immobilization of the ureter. Adequate peristalsis of the ureter also depends on normal function of the ureteral smooth muscle. Urinary tract **infection** may lead to release of bacterial endotoxin, resulting in loss of muscular contraction of the ureter and functional obstruction.

ABNORMAL DRAINAGE OF THE URETERS. Anatomic abnormalities inhibiting drainage of the ureters may also cause functional obstruction of the urinary tract. The ureters enter the bladder at the ureterovesical junction. Normally, the ureterovesical junction acts as a flap valve. Urine may flow freely from the ureter into the bladder, but bladder urine is prevented from going into the ureter. Abnormalities of the ureterovesical junction may allow urine to back up from the bladder into the ureters. This condition is called **reflux** or, more properly, vesicoureteral reflux. Reflux allows transmission of high pressures generated during voiding into the ureters and also leads to increased volumes of urine in the ureters. Both processes inhibit peristalsis and impair drainage of the ureters, leading to functional obstruction. This process may cause **hydronephrosis, or dilation of the upper urinary tract,** and renal impairment.

NEUROGENIC ABNORMALITIES. **Neurogenic abnormalities** affecting the lower urinary tract are important causes of functional obstruction of the urinary tract. Contraction and relaxation of the bladder must be closely integrated with appropriate relaxation and contraction of the urinary sphincter mechanisms to ensure the normal storage and voiding functions of the lower urinary tract. Impairment of these integrated functions may result from congenital or acquired lesions. Functional obstruction may result.

EFFECTS OF URINARY TRACT OBSTRUCTION

The Obstructive Process
In comparison to other excretory organs, the urinary tract has a most unusual response to obstruction. Other excretory organs stop functioning after obstruction.

In contrast, **the kidney and ureter continue to function after obstruction but develop hydronephrosis, a unique form of damage.**

After obstruction occurs glomerular function continues at a lower level. Furthermore, the filtered urine is changed by the processes of tubular reabsorption and secretion. In order to have continued urinary inflow, there must be some mechanism for outflow of urine by routes other than the ureter. Such outflow is provided by both the venous and the lymphatic systems. Therefore, **urine in the obstructed renal pelvis undergoes constant modification** as long as there is some functioning renal parenchyma.

The **extent of nephron damage depends on** a number of factors, that have been well defined in experimental systems. These factors include the **degree of obstruction** (complete or partial), the **duration of obstruction,** whether the process affects **one or both kidneys**, and the presence of associated urinary tract **infection.** In the clinical setting, however, it may be difficult to determine such factors as the duration of obstruction.

Hydronephrosis, the response of the upper urinary tract to obstruction, is associated with both anatomic and functional changes.

Anatomic Changes

Gross Pathology. For the first few weeks after complete obstruction of the ureter, there is progressive **dilation of the renal pelvis and ureter** above the site of obstruction. Due to accumulation of edema fluid, the weight of the kidney increases despite atrophy of the renal tissue. After 4 to 8 weeks of obstruction, the renal parenchymal weight decreases, since atrophy of the renal tissue exceeds the accumulation of edema fluid (Fig.12–2). At this time, the obstructed kidney is dark blue in color with scattered wedges of congestion and necrosis.

Microscopic Pathology. Microscopic changes are **first noted in the renal papillae and tubules.** During the first few days, there is flattening of the papillae and widespread dilation of the distal nephrons. The tubules dilate during the first few days of obstruction, then show progressive atrophy. In contrast, the glomeruli appear to be relatively resistant to obstructive injury. On light microscopic examination, pathologic changes are first noted after 4 weeks of obstruction. However, recent electron microscopic studies have shown that obstruction is accompanied by characteristic Tam-Horsfall protein casts within Bowman's space of the glomeruli. (Tam-Horsfall protein is synthesized only in the ascending limb of Henle's loop and the distal convoluted tubule.)

Obstructive uropathy also is accompanied by microscopic changes in the renal pelvis and ureter. Initially, there is hypertrophy of the smooth muscle proximal to the site of obstruction. Collagen and elastic tissue are then produced by the smooth muscle cells. This increase in connective tissue impairs transmission of peristaltic waves in the collecting system.

Functional Changes

Loss of renal function is the most important effect of obstructive uropathy. Animal models have proven to be especially valuable for determining the precise sequence of events following obstruction. Immediately after acute obstruction, there is a transient rise in renal blood flow. The increase in renal perfusion lasts for several hours and is followed by a progressive decrease in renal blood flow. The decrease in renal blood flow is due to the combination of active vasoconstriction and the initial elevation of ureteral pressure. Vasoconstriction appears to be the most important factor because ureteral pressure is soon reduced to near normal levels. Thus, **the two major factors responsible for nephron damage following obstruction appear to be ischemia and hydrostatic pressure.**

Obstruction is followed by a predictable sequence of adverse effects on renal function. Functional changes first affect the renal tubules and subsequently affect the glomeruli. **Ability to produce a concentrated urine is the first tubular function to fail after obstruction.** This is followed by an inability to acidify the urine and failure of proximal tubular secretory capacity. Glomerular function is preserved better than tubular function after obstruction. **Urinary dilution is the last renal function to be impaired** following obstruction. The amount of renal damage depends on both the completeness and the duration of obstruction. In addition, the presence of urinary tract infection greatly accelerates the rate of renal damage in an obstructed system. Eventually, all renal functions are lost.

Changes in the ureter accompany the renal changes following an obstructive injury. **Immediately after ureteral occlusion, there is an increase in both baseline and peak ureteral pressures** generated during peristalsis. The forceful contractions that result may cause marked elevation in the amplitude of the ureteral pressure waves and are responsible for the characteristic colic experienced by patients passing ureteral stones.

If obstruction persists, however, the increased ureteral force is used solely to counteract the increasing pressure within the ureteral lumen. This leads to persistent elevation in the baseline tension, with loss of peristalsis. With long-standing obstruction, there is decompensation of the ureteral wall, leading to dilation of the ureter, characteristic of obstruction. Decompensation also results in an increased ureteral volume and low pressure. Thus, **with chronic obstruction, the intraluminal pressure within the ureter is in the normal range.** The baseline tension in the ureter remains elevated because of the increased ureteral diameter (following LaPlace's law). Although the dilated ureter may still be able to generate contractions, the contractions will be decreased in magnitude and unable to close the ureteral walls. This leads to urine stasis, which predisposes to infection and stone formation.

FUNCTIONAL RECOVERY AFTER RELIEF OF OBSTRUCTION AND POSTOBSTRUCTIVE DIURESIS

Importance

Prompt diagnosis of obstructive uropathy is of critical importance because the cause of obstruction often is correctable and may lead to recovery of renal function. **The obstructed kidney has an amazing capacity for recovery of function**

following relief of obstruction. The ability of the obstructed kidney to recover function has been studied best in dogs. In this model system it is clear that **recovery is inversely related to the duration of obstruction.** Complete recovery is possible after 7 days of complete unilateral obstruction, but there is no recovery after 6 weeks of obstruction. Although it is usually difficult to determine the precise duration of obstruction in patients, clinical experience indicates that the human kidney may possess greater capacity for functional recovery than experimental animals. Recovery of some renal function has been documented in one patient after 69 days of complete ureteral obstruction. Other factors that influence the amount of functional recovery include the **severity of obstruction** and the presence of superimposed **infection.**

Nephron Recovery After Relief of Chronic Hydronephrosis

The pattern of recovery following relief of obstruction **depends on whether the process affects one or both kidneys.**

Unilateral Obstruction. With complete, unilateral obstruction of the upper urinary tract, **fluid and electrolyte balance remains normal, reflecting continued function of the contralateral, unobstructed kidney** Fig.12–2). There are none of the metabolic, hemodynamic, or hormonal changes characteristic of uremia. In all reported cases, there has been impairment of urinary concentrating ability with preserva-

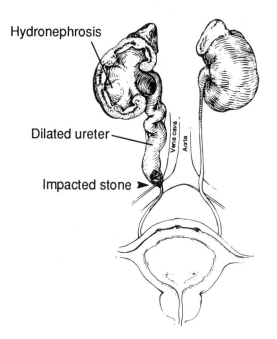

Hydronephrosis

Dilated ureter

Impacted stone ►

Vena cava

Aorta

Figure 12–2. Changes associated with unilateral hydronephrosis due to an obstructing right ureteral calculus. Because the patient has a normal left kidney, removal of the stone would not result in postobstructive diuresis. *(Modified from Tanagho EA, McAninch JW: Smith's General Urology, 12th ed. Norwalk, Conn: Appleton & Lange, 1988, p. 174.)*

tion of urinary dilution. Defects in all other aspects of renal function have been documented in individual patients, but there is no consistent pattern.

In animal studies, it has been shown that even mild, partial ureteral obstruction may significantly impair renal function. After relief of obstruction, there may be significant recovery of renal function in the presence of a normal, contralateral kidney. However, it has been shown that removing the normal kidney at the time that the obstruction is relieved leads to maximal recovery of function following unilateral obstruction.

Bilateral Obstruction (Or Obstruction of a Solitary Kidney). There are two major, clinically significant differences between unilateral and bilateral obstruction. First, bilateral ureteral obstruction may cause uremia, with all the complications discussed in Chapter 13. In contrast, unilateral obstruction does not cause uremia in the presence of a normal, contralateral kidney. Second, **release of bilateral obstruction is accompanied by a marked absolute and fractional loss of sodium (termed natriuresis) and water (termed diuresis)** (Fig.12–3). In contrast, relief of unilateral obstruction results in an increased fractional excretion of sodium and water (from the damaged kidney) but no absolute increase in excretion of salt and water. Short-lived, mild increases in urine output occur commonly after release of bilateral obstruction (or relief of obstruction in a solitary kidney). The diuresis is

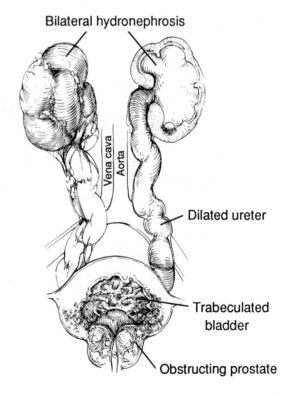

Figure 12–3. Bilateral hydronephrosis resulting from bladder neck obstruction by an enlarged prostate. Relief of obstruction may lead to postobstructive diuresis because both renal units are affected by the obstructive process. *(Modified from Tanagho EA, McAninch JW: Smith's General Urology, 12th ed. Norwalk, Conn: Appleton & Lange, 1988, p. 172.)*

physiologic, representing excretion of retained excess salt and water accumulated as a result of the previous obstruction.

Postobstructive Diuresis

Definition. **Copious urine output may occur following relief of urinary obstruction.** This process appears to result from **(1) decreased reabsorption of sodium, (2) a defect in urinary concentrating ability, (3) solute-induced diuresis, and (4) fluid overload that occurred during the period of obstruction.** The solute-induced diuresis is due to excretion of retained urea and may be prolonged by parenteral administration of glucose and salt.

Although it is unusual, **postobstructive diuresis may be life-threatening.** Therefore, any patient who has relief of obstruction should be closely monitored by following physical findings, particularly mental status, postural changes in blood pressure, hourly urine output, and daily weights. Laboratory studies should include close monitoring of serum and urine electrolytes and osmolarity.

Management. In practice, there is wide variation in the responses of patients following relief of bilateral obstruction. Mild diuresis and natriuresis are common and represent physiologic excretion of excess salt and water. In the presence of persistently high urinary output (greater than 200 ml/hour), the patient requires close monitoring. However, in the alert conscious patient, intravenous therapy generally is not necessary. **Given free access to fluids, the normal thirst mechanism usually will be adequate to restore fluid volume.** In this situation, overly vigorous administration of intravenous fluids and solutes (as is often practiced in clinical services) often prolongs the diuresis.

If the patient is comatose or immobile or if there is inappropriate sodium loss, approximately half of the urinary loss should be replaced by the intravenous route, with close monitoring of serum and urine chemistries.

SAMPLE ANSWERS TO STUDY QUESTIONS

1. Define obstructive uropathy and explain the significance of this condition.

Obstructive uropathy includes the pathologic effects of blockage on the anatomy and function of the urinary system. This is a common cause of morbidity and loss of renal function. Early diagnosis of obstructive uropathy is important because many of the causes are correctable. Correction of the underlying problem prevents further renal damage and may be accompanied by significant improvement in renal function.

2. Classify the potential causes of obstructive uropathy.

The causes of obstructive uropathy may be classified as either anatomic or functional problems.

Anatomic problems are areas of mechanical blockage. These problems may be subclassified as either congenital abnormalities, most common in children, or acquired abnormalities, most common in adults. Anatomic obstructions may also be considered as either intrinsic, meaning that the primary abnormality is within the urinary tract, or extrinsic, meaning that the primary problem is outside the urinary tract.

Functional abnormalities in transport of the urine may cause obstruction in the absence of anatomic blockage. The three mechanisms by which functional problems may cause obstruction are (1) abnormal peristalsis in the upper urinary tract, (2) abnormal drainage of the ureters, and (3) neurogenic abnormalities of the lower urinary tract.

3. Give two examples of each major cause of obstruction in Question 2.

    I. Anatomic–intrinsic obstructions
        A. Congenital anomalies
            1. Ureteropelvic junction obstruction
            2. Posterior urethral valves
        B. Acquired abnormalities
            1. Renal stone
            2. BPH
    II. Anatomic–extrinsic obstructions
        A. Retroperitoneal fibrosis
        B. Cancer arising from other organ (e.g., bowel, cervix, breast)
    III. Functional Obstructions
        A. Reflux
        B. Neurogenic bladder

4. Explain the effects of obstruction on the urinary tract.

The kidney and ureter continue to function after obstruction but become hydronephrotic. The extent of renal damage depends on many factors, including duration of obstruction, whether obstruction is unilateral or bilateral, the severity of obstruction (complete or partial), and the presence of superimposed infection. Obstructive uropathy is associated with anatomic and functional changes.

Dilation of the renal pelvis and of the ureter are the characteristic gross pathologic changes associated with obstruction. Microscopic changes are noted first in the renal tubules. The glomeruli are relatively resistant to the adverse effects of obstruction of the urinary tract.

Decreased function of both the kidney and ureter accompanies obstructive uropathy. Loss of renal function is the most important change. Tubular functions are most sensitive to obstructive injury. Ability to produce a concentrated urine is the first tubular function to fail, and urinary dilution is the renal function most resistant to obstructive injury. After obstruction, the ureter eventually loses the ability to generate an effective peristaltic wave for transport of the urinary stream.

5. Explain the nature and significance of postobstructive diuresis.

The obstructed kidney has a remarkable capacity to recover function after relief of obstruction. Occasionally, brisk and prolonged diuresis may occur after relief of bilateral obstruction or relief of obstruction of a solitary kidney. This is called postobstructive diuresis. Four factors may contribute to this process: (1) decreased reabsorption of sodium, (2) defective urinary concentration, (3) solute-induced diuresis, and (4) retention of excess fluids accumulated during the time the urinary tract was obstructed. Occurrence of postobstructive diuresis is cause for concern and is an indication for close patient monitoring because this condition may be life-threatening. However, vigorous intravenous fluid replacement generally is unnecessary in alert patients given free access to liquids, since the normal thirst mechanism usually is adequate to restore fluid volume.

Chronic Renal Failure

Management of Severe CRF and ESRD
  General considerations
  Dialysis
  Transplantation
SAMPLE ANSWERS TO STUDY QUESTIONS

INTRODUCTION

Chronic renal failure is a common cause of renal failure and death. Each year between 50 and 150 persons per million population require dialysis or renal transplantation or die of renal failure. Thus, at any given time, a large number of patients are suffering the consequences of chronic renal failure.

STUDY QUESTIONS

1. How does chronic renal failure differ from end-stage renal disease?
2. **a.** Classify the causes of chronic renal failure.
   b. What is the most common cause of chronic renal failure in the United States?
   c. What is the most important, treatable cause of chronic renal failure among black Americans?
3. **a.** At what level of renal function is replacement therapy necessary?
   b. List the available types of renal replacement therapy.
4. **a.** Classify the four major categories of clinical manifestations of chronic renal failure.
   b. Give one example for each category in Question a.
5. Give three reasons why early diagnosis of chronic renal failure is important.
6. **a.** What is the significance of kidney size?
   b. What clinical method can be used to determine the kidney size?
7. Is blood urea nitrogen (BUN) concentration a reliable indicator of renal function?
8. List five reversible conditions that can aggravate renal failure.
9. List the most important factors in bone metabolism in patients with chronic renal failure.

DEFINITION AND CAUSES OF CHRONIC RENAL FAILURE

Definitions

Chronic Renal Failure (CRF). The term chronic renal failure suggests **chronic and generally irreversible failure of renal function.** Usually, the course of CRF is progressive. In other words, the renal function gradually gets worse. **With proper management, the course of CRF can sometimes be modified and, in occasional cases, reversed.**

End-Stage Renal Disease (ESRD). **When renal function deteriorates to a point where either dialysis or transplantation becomes necessary to sustain life,** it is called end-stage renal disease. **ESRD is not reversible.**

Causes

Numerous renal and systemic diseases can cause CRF. The most common causes are listed in Table 13–1.

CLINICAL MANIFESTATIONS

The symptoms and signs of renal failure are extremely variable. This is true in two respects. First, the clinical manifestations may be very different among different patients with similar degrees of renal insufficiency. Second, the symptoms and signs of renal failure may be very different in the same patient at different times. Table 13–2 outlines the clinical manifestations of renal failure at various stages of progression.

The key clinical index of renal function is the **creatinine clearance**, which estimates the glomerular filtration rate (GFR). The normal creatinine clearance is 100 to 120 mL/min. **Symptoms of renal failure generally become evident when the GFR, as measured by creatinine clearance, falls below 20–30 mL/min.** Thus, there may be very few symptoms and signs of renal disease until more than 80% of the renal function has been lost. **Severe manifestations occur once the GFR reaches 10 mL/min.** At this level of renal function, the patient requires either **dialysis or transplantation** to survive. These treatments are collectively called **renal replacement therapy.**

The most common signs and symptoms of renal failure include general

TABLE 13–1. COMMON CAUSES OF CHRONIC RENAL FAILURE

Type of Disorder	Example
Glomerulonephritis (GN) (most common cause of ESRD in USA)	Rapidly progressive GN Mesangioproliferative GN Focal segmental GN
Systemic diseases	Diabetes Vasculitis Lupus erythematosus
Hypertension (especially in black Americans)	Any cause
Nephrotoxins	Analgesics Antibiotics
Genetic disorders	Polycystic kidney disease Alport's syndrome (congenital deafness + CRF)
Urologic disorders	Obstructive nephropathy Stones Tumors

TABLE 13–2. CLINICAL MANIFESTATIONS OF PROGRESSING RENAL FAILURE

Creatinine Clearance (mL/min)	Symptoms	Physical Findings	Laboratory Results
>35	None	Hypertension, common	Hct 30–40
20–35	Fatigue, anorexia, cramps, nocturia	All of above ± edema	Hct 25–35 ± acidosis, hyperphosphatemia
10–20	All of above + nausea ± itching, edema, olfactory abnormal, arthritis[a]	All of above ± ecchymoses, pericarditis, arthritis	All of above worsen + hypocalcemia
<10	All of above worsen + vomiting paresthesis ± seizures, coma	All above worsen	All above worsen

[a] +, in addition; ±, common but not inevitable.

malaise, lack of energy, easy fatigability, unexplained normochromic normocytic anemia (also termed anemia of chronic disease), fluid excess, hypertension, and nocturia. Symptoms that occur later include itching, nausea, vomiting, and disturbances of smell and taste. With better management and early institution of dialysis, severe acidosis, uremic frost, pericarditis, uremic lungs, and various neurologic manifestations, which formerly typified the uremic patient, are rare.

The clinical manifestations of renal failure reflect four fundamental pathologic processes: (1) loss of renal exocrine functions, (2) loss of renal endocrine functions, (3) hyperparathyroidism, and (4) uremia.

Loss of Renal Exocrine Function
Loss of exocrine function reflects reduction in the number of functioning nephrons and causes changes in the internal environment.

Sodium Handling. Because of loss of functioning nephrons, the normal salt load cannot be removed by the kidney. Until GFR declines to about 30 mL/min, the fractional excretion of sodium (percent of filtered Na excreted) is kept constant by an ill-defined mechanism termed glomerulotubular feedback. The fractional excretion of sodium increases when GFR is reduced below 30 mL/min. In other words, proportionally more filtered Na is lost in the urine. Thus, the damaged kidney tries to maintain sodium balance by markedly increasing its fractional excretion in the face of declining nephron function. This relationship is illustrated in Figure 13–1. As more nephrons are lost, sodium retention becomes inevitable. The two common consequences of sodium retention are (1) extracellular volume (ECV) excess, manifested by edema, elevated jugular venous pressure, and so on, and (2) hypertension, with its complications (e.g., left ventricular hypertrophy, headaches, atherosclerosis, further renal damage).

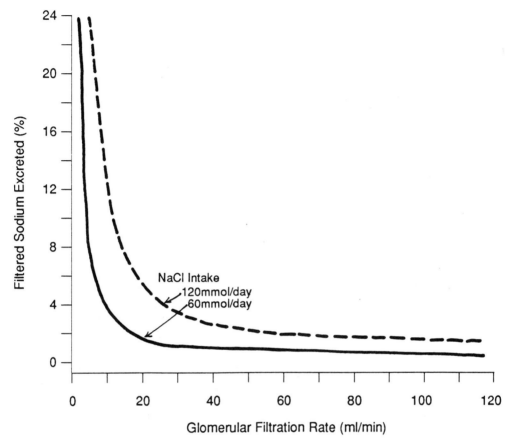

Figure 13–1. Fractional excretion of sodium with varying renal function.

Water. Loss of functioning nephrons limits the ability of the kidney to regulate water metabolism. **Eventually, the damaged kidney is unable to either concentrate or dilute the urine.** Thus, excessive water intake may result in dilution of plasma (hyponatremia, water excess) due to inability to excrete a dilute urine. On the other hand, insufficient water intake quickly leads to water depletion (hypernatremia) due to inability to concentrate the urine. Water depletion is unusual in otherwise normal individuals because of thirst.

Potassium Regulation. **With a normal potassium intake, the kidney usually is able to prevent hyperkalemia until the GFR declines below 10 mL/min.** Beyond this point, potassium restriction may be necessary to prevent the potentially fatal complications of hyperkalemia. Patients with diabetic nephropathy or interstitial diseases, who have type 4 renal tubular acidosis, tend to develop hyperkalemia earlier than other patients with similar degrees of renal insufficiency. In addition, patients with less severe reductions of GFR may develop hyperkalemia if potassium intake is excessive or if potassium excretion is altered by drugs.

Acid-Base Regulation. Renal failure causes retention of hydrogen ion produced by cellular metabolism. This leads to **metabolic acidosis.** Concurrently, the unmeasured anions also are retained. Thus, there is an **increase in the anion gap.**

Phosphate Retention. With declining GFR, phosphate excretion is reduced in the urine. Therefore, the level of phosphate increases in the bloodstream. **Phosphate retention contributes to bone disease**, so-called **renal osteodystrophy,** in patients with CRF.

Loss of Renal Endocrine Function

All three major renal endocrine functions are affected in patients with renal insufficiency. Thus, there are changes in (1) vitamin D metabolism, (2) erythropoietin secretion, and (3) renin secretion.

Vitamin D Metabolism. Vitamin D is changed to its active form $(1,25(OH)_2D_3)$ by functioning renal tissue. With the loss of renal parenchyma, there is a **relative deficiency** of this active form of vitamin D. This leads to **poor calcium absorption** that further aggravates the metabolic bone disease.

Erythropoietin. **Erythropoietin** is the key hormone that **regulates production of red blood cells by the bone marrow.** Because erythropoietin is produced only in the kidney, loss of functioning renal parenchyma causes a deficiency of this hormone. **Erythropoietin deficiency is the major factor contributing to the anemia of renal failure.**

Renin Excess. Renin is another hormone that is produced by the kidney. This hormone is important in the regulation of blood pressure. **In 10 to 15% of patients with chronic renal failure, hypertension is caused by an increased release of renin from the damaged kidney.**

Compensation to Renal Parenchymal Loss (Hyperparathyroidism)

Hypocalcemia and vitamin D deficiency stimulate the parathyroid glands. This leads to increased production of parathyroid hormone (PTH). Because the primary disorder is in the kidney, not the parathyroid, this is classified as a form of secondary hyperparathyroidism. Since the kidney is a major site of PTH metabolism, kidney failure also prolongs the half-life of PTH, compounding the problem.

Uremia

Retention of known (e.g., acid, urea, creatinine) and unknown metabolic products contributes to a variety of clinical manifestations in patients with renal failure. Some of the most common include anorexia, nausea, vomiting, serositis, and neuropathy. This constellation of clinical findings is termed uremia.

The exact pathogenesis of the uremic syndrome is not known. It is likely that the clinical manifestations of uremia are caused by retained metabolic products. In addition, deficiency of erythropoietin causes anemia, and deficiency of active vitamin D aggravates renal osteodystrophy. Hyperparathyroidism may contribute to uremic symptoms.

DIAGNOSIS OF CHRONIC RENAL FAILURE (CRF)

Importance of Early Diagnosis of CRF

Symptoms of renal failure appear late in the course of CRF, usually after 80% or more of functioning renal tissue has been lost. At the time of diagnosis, most patients with CRF have no prior history of preexisting renal disease. Thus, **the majority of patients with CRF at any given time are in the silent pre-ESRD phase.**

There are two reasons why the early diagnosis of CRF is important. First, it may be possible to identify a reversible cause of renal dysfunction. For example, removal of obstructing prostatic tissue may prevent permanent renal damage. Second, the rate of progression of renal failure sometimes can be slowed by early diagnosis and appropriate management. Protein restriction or some medications may modify the rate of progression in all forms of CRF. Treatment of rapidly progressive glomerulonephritis with immunosuppression or plasma exchange can reverse or slow the rate of renal deterioration. Therefore, **early diagnosis of CRF offers the opportunity to substantially change the course and outcome of the disease process.**

General Considerations in Diagnosis

Determining renal size and monitoring renal function are two critical considerations in the management of any patient with CRF.

Kidney Size. Finding that the kidneys are already small in size means that most functioning tissue has been replaced by fibrous tissue. Thus, there is likely to be little reversibility of the renal failure. Examination of the kidneys with ultrasound is usually the optimal way to determine renal size. In an average size adult, kidneys less than 7.5 cm in size with thin cortical tissue are usually not amenable to specific therapy. In contrast, finding normal or enlarged kidneys means that additional studies are needed to delineate a potentially reversible cause of renal failure.

Monitoring Renal Function. The loss of functioning nephrons is proportional to the decline in GFR. For sophisticated physiologic studies, GFR is determined by calculating inulin clearance (see Chapter 2). **Measurement of serum creatinine and creatinine clearance are the standard clinical tests for estimating renal function (GFR).** Creatinine is a by-product of muscle metabolism and is freely filtered at the glomerulus. Clearance of creatinine closely correlates with GFR and is clinically used to follow renal function. Generation of creatinine usually is constant and is proportional to muscle mass. Under most conditions, creatinine removal is carried out mainly by the kidney. The serum creatinine concentration will largely depend on GFR. **There is an inverse relationship between serum creatinine and creatinine clearance (GFR): serum creatinine increases as creatinine clearance goes down.** Thus, serum creatinine is also useful in following renal function. The normal serum creatinine concentration is about 1 mg/dL.

In some situations, serum creatinine concentration may not be an accurate reflection of reduced renal function. For example, in advanced uremia, creatinine generation may be reduced due to muscle wasting, creatinine secretion by the renal tubule may increase, and extrarenal metabolism of creatinine (mainly in the gut) also increases. Thus, renal function may be significantly worse than the serum creatinine level suggests. There are also limitations to the use of creatinine clearance as an estimate of renal function. Recently, it has been shown that creatinine clearance overestimates GFR (as determined by inulin clearance). As GFR declines, this difference between creatinine clearance and inulin clearance becomes more pronounced. Despite these limitations, serum creatinine and creatinine clearance are the standard clinical methods for determining and monitoring GFR. Measurement of creatinine clearance requires collection of urine over 24 hours, plus a simultaneous blood specimen for determination of the serum creatinine concentration.

Measurement of the concentration of blood urea nitrogen (BUN) also is used clinically to estimate renal function. Urea is produced by metabolism of dietary protein, and its removal depends on the balance between filtration at the glomerulus (GFR) and tubular reabsorption. (The normal ratio of BUN to serum creatinine is about 20:1.) **The problem with the use of BUN as a measure of renal function is that BUN concentration depends on factors other than GFR.** For example, the state of hydration or changes in protein intake would alter the BUN. In addition, BUN may be increased in some pathologic situations, whereas GFR remains constant. For example, gastrointestinal tract hemorrhage may lead to an increase in BUN with no change in renal function due to hypovolemia, with decreased GFR and increased tubular reabsorption of urea. **Thus, BUN is not a reliable clinical indicator of renal function.**

MANAGEMENT OF CRF

A systematic approach to management of patients with CRF includes consideration of three broad areas. First, there are general factors that must be considered in every patient. Second, there are specific problems that require management in selected patients. Third, renal replacement therapy, that is, dialysis and transplantation, can now be considered routinely in almost all patients with severe renal insufficiency.

General Considerations in All Patients with CRF

Identify Reversible Factors. In chronically diseased kidneys, renal function can be further compromised by several potentially reversible factors. Therefore, **the first step in any patient with CRF is to identify potentially reversible factors that contribute to renal dysfunction.** There are four common, reversible causes of CRF: **(1) hypoperfusion, (2) obstruction, (3) nephrotoxins, and (4) infection.** There are also other less common, reversible factors that may need to be considered in some patients with CRF.

Hypoperfusion may lead to decreased renal function. Kidneys may be underperfused as a result of extracellular fluid (ECF) depletion secondary to overzealous use of diuretics or because of heart failure. Hypoperfusion causes a further decline in GFR, with increased renal tubular reabsorption of the glomerular filtrate, particularly urea. Creatinine is not reabsorbed. Thus, **renal function deteriorates suddenly, with a disproportionate increase in BUN relative to the increase in serum creatinine.**

Hypoperfusion is suggested by a number of clinical findings. These include orthostatic changes in blood pressure and heart rate, signs of congestive failure, increased BUN to creatinine ratio (>20:1), and decreased urinary sodium excretion (fractional excretion of sodium ≤ 1%). Restoration of renal perfusion is the optimal therapy. For ECF depletion, discontinuation of diuretics may be sufficient to improve renal perfusion. In severe cases, however, liberalization of salt intake, or even careful intravenous infusion of saline may be required. Treatment of congestive cardiac failure, if present, also may improve renal function.

Any cause of **obstruction at any site along the urinary tract** may further aggravate renal failure. Sonography is a useful, noninvasive technique to help rule out significant obstruction in most cases. This technique may be misleading in some patients with incomplete obstruction or in certain diseases that limit the ability of the collecting system to expand.* If possible, intravenous contrast studies should be avoided because of the nephrotoxicity of radiographic contrast media, particularly in patients with diabetes.

Nephrotoxic agents often aggravate CRF. The three most common nephrotoxins are **nonsteroidal anti-inflammatory drugs, aminoglycoside antibiotics, and contrast media.** Deterioration of renal function associated with administration of these agents usually is reversible if recognized early and the offending agent is discontinued. Nephrotoxicity associated with drug administration occurs most often in patients with other risk factors. These factors include previously impaired renal function, diabetes mellitus, nephrotic syndrome, old age, and severe heart disease.

Deterioration of renal function has been reported following excretory urography, angiography, cholecystography, and computed tomography. Administration of contrast media is particularly risky in patients with Bence-Jones nephropathy or with diabetic nephropathy. If contrast media is necessary in pa-

---

*For example, scarring from previous surgery, or retroperitoneal carcinomatosis.

tients with CRF, the use of a minimal dose, volume expansion, and the infusion of mannitol (an osmotic diuretic) before and after the procedure will maintain good urine flow and may reduce the risk of nephrotoxicity.

Certain drugs, such as diuretics, antibiotics (i.e., sulfonamides, methacillin), and allopurinol, cause interstitial nephritis. Such drugs with a high risk of causing renal problems should be avoided in patients with compromised renal function.

Uncomplicated lower **urinary tract infections** do not cause renal damage. In contrast, upper urinary tract infections may cause renal scarring. **Loss of renal function is especially rapid when infection occurs in an obstructed kidney.** In patients with underlying renal disease, any additional compromise of renal function may exacerbate uremia. Therefore, diagnosis of urinary tract infection, appropriate antibacterial therapy, and correction of underlying anatomic causes are important for the preservation of renal function.

A number of **other reversible factors** may contribute to renal insufficiency. Three factors to be considered include **hypercalcemia, renal vein thrombosis, and pregnancy.** Hypercalcemia (serum calcium >12 mg/dL) may worsen renal function. Renal vein thrombosis may cause sudden deterioration of renal function in a nephrotic patient. This is especially likely to be the case if there is evidence of other thromboembolic problems. Anticoagulation is indicated if the diagnosis of renal vein thrombosis is confirmed with radiologic studies. Pregnancy may result in further deterioration of renal function in patients with CRF. Women with compromised renal function should be warned about this possibility. If pregnancy occurs, renal function should be monitored carefully, and blood pressure should be controlled to prevent further deterioration of renal function.

Control Hypertension. More than 80% of patients with a GFR below 30 mL/min have elevated blood pressure. **Control of hypertension is the single most important factor influencing the rate of progression of renal failure.** Good control of blood pressure reduces the rate at which renal function deteriorates. This effect is especially well documented in patients with diabetic nephropathy. Initially, lowering of blood pressure may be associated with a transient decline in renal function. **Despite this possibility of transient worsening of renal function, elevated blood pressure should always be treated, since the hazards of uncontrolled hypertension exceed those of transient worsening of renal function.**

Apart from influencing the rate of progression of renal failure, uncontrolled hypertension also is the single most important factor causing **accelerated atherosclerosis** in patients with CRF. Complications of atherosclerosis are major causes of death and morbidity in patients with CRF and ESRD. Therefore, control of hypertension is critical in the patient's overall treatment regimen.

Most hypertensive patients with CRF have ECF excess. Consequently, **limitation of dietary salt intake** and the use of **diuretics** are usually the first steps in the treatment of hypertension. If the GFR is <30 mL/min, milder diuretics usually are not effective, and loop diuretics, such as furosemide, are necessary. **Potassium-sparing diuretics and potassium supplements usually are contraindicated because of the risk of hyperkalemia.**

If diuretics alone are not effective, vasodilators, such as hydralazine, calcium channel blockers, such as nifedipine and minoxidil, or beta-blockers, such as metoprolol, can be added to the treatment regimen. Drugs that are metabolized by the kidney, such as atenolol and pindolol, may accumulate in patients with renal failure. These agents should be used with caution and dose adjustment. Recently, angiotensin-converting enzyme inhibitors, like captopril and enalapril, have been said to be useful in slowing the rate of progression of renal failure, particularly in patients with diabetic nephropathy. They presumably reduce the intraglomerular pressure, thereby slowing the progression of glomerulosclerosis. More work is needed to further define the role of these drugs in CRF.

Modify Diet. **Limitation of the intake of dietary protein leads to improvement of uremic symptoms.** With the availability of dialysis, and because of concern about the potential for development of protein malnutrition, use of severe protein restriction became controversial and passed from favor. This controversy has recently shown a new wrinkle. In animal work and a few human studies, **moderate protein restriction has been shown to slow the progression of renal failure.** The theoretical explanation is that ingestion of excessive protein leads to excess filtration by individual, functioning glomeruli in patients with CRF. Persistent hyperfiltration leads to progressive sclerosis of the remaining glomeruli. Intake of a low protein diet has been proposed to reduce the severity of glomerular hyperfiltration, thereby slowing the progression of glomerulosclerosis. More studies are needed to validate this hypothesis. More importantly, additional studies are needed to establish that protein restriction is safe and does not cause malnutrition or tissue loss.

With advancing renal failure (GFR <20 mL/min), **other dietary restrictions** may be necessary. If ECF excess is present, sodium should be restricted to about 60 mEq a day. If serum potassium rises the daily allowance of potassium should not exceed 60 mEq. Hyperphosphatemia is usually handled by restricting dairy products and the use of oral phosphate binders. Most patients maintain good water balance with the daily allowance of total water limited to between 1000 and 2000 mL.

Specific Considerations

Renal Osteodystrophy. This bone disease in patients with CRF, reflects profound changes in calcium and phosphate metabolism. There are four primary defects in calcium metabolism in patients with CRF: (1) renal retention of phosphorus, (2) reduced levels of active vitamin D, (3) reduced calcium intake, and (4) hyperparathyroidism (Fig. 13–2).

Renal retention of phosphorus causes hyperphosphatemia (increased serum levels of phosphates). Because of the reciprocal relationship between serum phosphate and serum calcium, hyperphosphatemia causes a reduction in serum calcium.

Reduced levels of active vitamin D. Renal parenchyma activates vitamin D to 1,25-dihydroxyvitamin D_3 [1,25 $(OH)_2D_3$], the most active form. With loss of renal

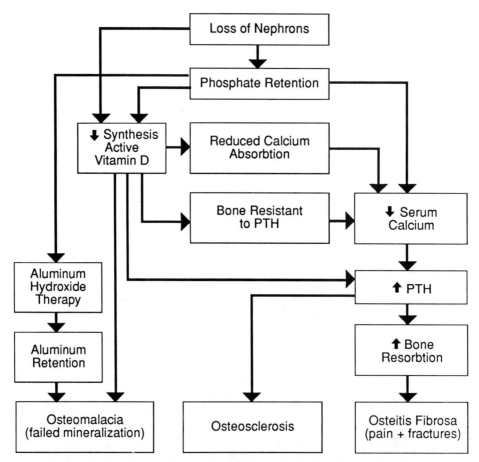

Figure 13–2. Interaction of hormones and minerals in the etiology of renal osteodystrophy.

parenchyma, the synthesis of 1,25 $(OH)_2D_3$ is reduced. Dihydroxyvitamin D_3 has three effects: it enhances gut absorption, it increases bone mineral resorption, and it inhibits parathyroid hormone. All of these effects are impaired in patients with renal failure. The net effect is a further reduction of serum calcium.

Reduced intake of dietary calcium. As patients become anorectic (experience loss of appetite), they may reduce the intake of calcium-containing foods, resulting in more profound hypocalcemia.

Secondary hyperparathyroidism is common in patients with CRF. Hypocalcemia (low serum calcium) stimulates the parathyroid glands to secrete PTH. PTH usually stimulates resorption of bone. However, in uremia, bones are relatively resistant to PTH, and serum Ca does not increase proportionately.

In summary, patients with CRF tend to develop hyperphosphatemia, relative hypocalcemia, and hyperparathyroidism.

As GFR declines below 30, serum phosphate starts increasing, and serum calcium may decline. If the product of the serum calcium and serum phosphate is higher than 55, there is a risk that these **minerals may precipitate in soft tissues** (so-called **metastatic calcification**). Treatment involves a two-step process. First, the serum phosphate concentration should be lowered (below 6 mg/dL). Then calcium supplements are used if necessary. Hyperphosphatemia is controlled by restricting intake of dairy products and prescribing aluminum hydroxide antacids, which bind phosphate in the gut, preventing absorption. Until recently, the principal phosphate-binding antacid used was aluminum hydroxide. The demonstration that aluminum is quite toxic has led to the use of calcium carbonate and calcium acetate as the primary choices for phosphate control.

Serum calcium and phosphate levels should be monitored closely in patients with CRF to limit the potential development of metastatic calcification in soft tissues.

Metabolic Acidosis. **With severe renal failure, the usual daily excretion of 60 to 80 mEq of H$^+$ is impaired.** This results in positive H$^+$ balance and metabolic acidosis. The kidney also loses the ability to excrete unmeasured anions, such as HPO$_4^-$, resulting in accumulation of these anions and an **increase in the anion gap.**

A second type of metabolic acidosis may occur in patients with milder renal failure. Metabolic acidosis in these cases results from a tubular defect termed **renal tubular acidosis.** Renal tubular acidosis is associated with a normal anion gap.

Acidosis is well tolerated until the serum bicarbonate (HCO$_3^-$) drops below 15 mEq/L. If necessary, 20 to 40 mEq of sodium bicarbonate (NaHCO$_3$) or sodium citrate (Shohl's solution) a day is used to treat the acidosis. In the presence of hypertension or ECF excess, these sodium salts should be used cautiously. With the use of citrate solution, two points should be considered. First, only sodium citrate (not Na–K citrate) should be used to avoid hyperkalemia. Second, there is increasing evidence that citrate causes excessive absorption of aluminum and an increased risk of aluminum intoxication. Consequently, concomitant administration of citrate and aluminum should be avoided.

Anemia, Hyperkalemia, and Hyperuricemia. Anemia is common in patients with advanced renal failure and usually is multifactorial in origin. **Reduced synthesis of erythropoietin by the diseased kidney is probably the most important contributing factor.** Other treatable causes of anemia (such as nutritional deficiency or excessive blood loss) should be ruled out. Recombinant human erythropoietin recently has been proven effective in dialysis patients and is now available as therapy.

The renal tubules have a remarkable capacity to secrete potassium. Thus, **hyperkalemia (increased serum potassium) is uncommon until the terminal stages of renal failure.** An exception occurs in patients with one form of renal tubular acidosis who have an impaired capacity to handle potassium and can easily develop life-threatening hyperkalemia. Dietary potassium restriction, avoiding potassium-sparing diuretics and potassium salts usually can prevent this problem.

Hyperuricemia (increased serum uric acid) also is common in CRF. Uric acid values under 11 mg/dL seldom cause clinical problems. Allopurinol is used for patients with overt gout or those with higher uric acid levels.

Drug Dosage Modifications. Four general principles should be remembered when prescribing any medication for patients with CRF: (1) changes in drug metabolism, (2) increased risk of nephrotoxicity, (3) increased risk of hyperkalemia, and (4) potential side effects.

Changes in Drug Metabolism. If a drug or its active metabolites are eliminated by the kidney, the dose should be adjusted appropriately. The penicillins, aminoglycosides, digitalis preparations, and insulin are noteworthy examples.

Nephrotoxicity. Certain drugs, such as aminoglycoside antibiotics and nonsteroidal anti-inflammatory agents, have the potential to produce further renal damage. These drugs should either be avoided or used with caution in patients with CRF.

Hyperkalemia. Drugs, such as potassium supplements, potassium-sparing diuretics, and salt substitutes, can cause life-threatening hyperkalemia in patients with impaired renal function.

Side Effects. Certain side effects of drugs are more common in the presence of renal failure. Examples of side effects that are more common in patients with CRF include peripheral neuropathy from nitrofurantoins, digitalis toxicity, and ototoxicity and nephrotoxicity from aminoglycosides.

Vascular Access. Preservation of arm veins for later creation of vascular access for hemodialysis is one of the most important considerations in the management of patients with CRF. Unfortunately, this is often ignored. The result may be very difficult problems with vascular access when the patient reaches ESRD. **Forearm veins in patients with CRF should not be used for infusions, transfusions, or diagnostic venipunctures.** If possible, veins in the wrist, leg, or central veins should be used. Two to four months before initiation of dialysis, an arteriovenous fistula should be created. This ensures adequate time for the fistula vein to mature.

Psychosocial Aspects. Patients with CRF must make drastic adjustments in almost all aspects of everyday life. The patient, spouse, and family should be given details of the various aspects of the disease and its management in simple and clear terms. These discussions should be carried out in a relaxed, sympathetic, and nonthreatening fashion. It is better to see the patient and family frequently, with continued discussion in a frank and friendly atmosphere. Younger patients take longer to make the necessary changes in lifestyle and need more psychologic support. At an appropriate time, exposure to other well-adjusted and well-informed patients with ESRD is often very helpful. Group therapy and counseling may be beneficial.

Management of Severe CRF and ESRD

General Considerations. **Definitive therapy usually is necessary for treatment of uremic symptoms, fluid overload, hyperkalemia, or severe acidosis, when the BUN is above 100 mg/dL (normal <20) and the creatinine is above 6 to 8 mg/dL (normal≤1).** Patients with diabetic nephropathy often require dialysis earlier in the course of their disease.

Once a patient has reached ESRD, there are three choices: protein restriction plus palliative treatment, dialysis, and transplantation. It is important to have an ongoing discussion about these alternatives, especially the various considerations involved with the dialysis and transplant options, well before ESRD is reached. The third choice of doing nothing except diet restriction is hardest for the family and physician to accept, since it means eventual death for the patient. However, if the patient is terminally ill with other incurable conditions and makes a well-informed decision not to receive dialysis, this decision should be honored.

Dialysis. Removal of uremic toxins by artificial means had been investigated for over 75 years. However, up to 30 years ago, patients with renal failure had but one outlook, death with uremia. In 1960, Dr. Scribner and his colleagues at the University of Washington successfully dialyzed the first patient with ESRD. This pioneering effort was successful mainly because they had developed methods to maintain long-term vascular access. During the last 25 years, the growth of the population of patients on dialysis and the survival of these patients has exceeded the most optimistic expectations. In the United States, over 100,000 patients are alive on renal replacement therapy, and worldwide, this figure is approaching 250,000 patients.

The dialysis process simply involves transfer of solutes and water between the patient and a physiologic electrolyte solution, called dialysis fiuid, across a semipermeable membrane. In broad terms, two types of dialysis therapy are available, hemodialysis and peritoneal dialysis.

Hemodialysis. **During hemodialysis, blood is passed through a cartridge (dialyzer), where it is separated from a rinsing fluid (dialysate) by a semipermeable membrane.** The procedure usually lasts about 4 hours and is repeated three times per week. Predialysis BUN and creatinine concentrations generally are in the range of 80 to 100 and 8 to 14 mg/dL, respectively. ECF volume is controlled by ultrafiltration of plasma across the dialyzer membrane. Patients either can dialyze at outpatient units or can be trained to dialyze at home. Home dialysis is less expensive and allows a more normal lifestyle for the patient. These patients are generally healthier than patients who have dialysis at centers.

With dialysis, control of hypertension usually is straightforward, and uremic symptoms, such as vomiting and neuropathy, improve dramatically. Other problems, such as osteodystrophy, anemia, cardiovascular disease, and sexual problems, persist and require continued attention. Survival of hemodialysis patients has improved over the last decade. The leading cause of death is atherosclerosis and its complications. **Control of hypertension and cessation of smoking greatly improve survival.**

Peritoneal Dialysis. Intermittent cycling of dialysate into and out of the peritoneal cavity through an implanted catheter is called peritoneal dialysis. **The peritoneum functions as the dialysis membrane.** The procedure commonly involves infusion of 2 L of sterile dialysate into the peritoneal cavity from a plastic bag, then draining it out after about 6 hours. The cycle is repeated four times throughout a 24 hour period, and the procedure is called continuous ambulatory peritoneal dialysis. Continuous ambulatory peritoneal dialysis has to be performed around the clock every day. An alternative is to let an automated system (a cycler) cycle 2 L of fluid every 2 to 3 hours at night while the patient is sleeping. In some patients, the dialysis fluid is left in the peritoneal cavity during the daytime, a process called continuous cycling peritoneal dialysis.

There are several problems with peritoneal dialysis. Peritonitis is a major complication with both continuous ambulatory peritoneal dialysis and continuous cycling peritoneal dialysis. Peritoneal dialysis provides less overall clearance of solutes than does hemodialysis. Thus, for patients with a large dialysis requirement (e.g., a large man with no GFR), peritoneal dialysis may be inadequate to maintain well-being. The overall dropout rate for patients on peritoneal dialysis is also much higher than for patients on hemodialysis.

Transplantation. **A successful renal transplant provides a better quality of life than either peritoneal dialysis or hemodialysis.** However, the **limited availability** of cadaveric kidneys, surgical risks, side effects of immunosuppression, bone disease, and rejection of transplanted kidneys are major problems with this form of renal replacement therapy. Both living related donor and cadaveric transplants are carried out successfully. Rejection episodes and immunosuppression-related problems occur less often with organs from living related donors than with cadaveric organs. Newly available immunosuppressive agents (e.g., cyclosporine) have greatly improved the survival of renal transplants.

The three specific forms of renal replacement therapy are mutually complimentary and can be used according to patients' preferences and needs. For example, it is common for patients to start on dialysis therapy, then undergo transplantation if an appropriately matched kidney becomes available. If rejection of the renal graft occurs, peritoneal dialysis or hemodialysis is again employed. The development of safe and effective renal replacement therapies allows the physician to offer several alternatives to death for patients with severe renal failure and ESRD.

SAMPLE ANSWERS TO STUDY QUESTIONS

1. How does chronic renal failure differ from end-stage renal disease?

Chronic renal failure is the presence of long-standing, progressive, and generally irreversible deterioration of renal function. End-stage renal disease is the terminal phase of chronic renal failure, when either dialysis or transplantation is necessary to sustain life.

2. a. Classify the causes of chronic renal failure.

Primary glomerulonephritis

Systemic diseases (e.g. diabetes)

Hypertension

Nephrotoxins

Genetic disorders

Urologic diseases

b. What is the most common cause of chronic renal failure in the United States?

Primary glomerulonephritis

c. What is the most important, treatable cause of chronic renal failure among black Americans?

Hypertension

3. a. At what level of renal function is replacement therapy necessary?

GFR < 10 ml/min

b. List the available types of renal replacement therapy.

Dialysis
  Hemodialysis
  Peritoneal dialysis
    Continuous ambulatory peritoneal dialysis
    Continuous cycling peritoneal dialysis

Transplantation
  Living related donor transplantation
  Cadaveric donor transplantation

4. a. Classify the four major categories of clinical manifestations of chronic renal failure.

Loss of renal exocrine function

Loss of renal endocrine function

Compensation to renal parenchymal loss

Uremia

b. Give one example for each of categories in Question a.

Loss of renal exocrine function: ECV excess and hypertension

Loss of renal endocrine function: Vitamin D deficiency

Compensation to renal parenchymal loss: Hyperparathyroidism

Uremia: Nausea and vomiting

5. Give three reasons why early diagnosis of chronic renal failure is important.

With early diagnosis, the rate of progression of chronic renal failure may be slowed.

Reversible causes of renal failure, such as obstruction, can be eliminated.

Specific treatment may be instituted, such as immunosuppression for rapidly progressive renal failure.

6. a. What is the significance of kidney size?

The presence of normal sized kidneys should prompt further evaluation to identify, and possibly treat, reversible causes of renal failure. The presence of bilaterally small kidneys suggests that the renal damage is irreversible.

b. What clinical method can be used to determine the kidney size?

Ultrasound

7. Is blood urea nitrogen (BUN) concentration a reliable indicator of renal function?

No. BUN can change secondary to extrarenal factors, such as protein intake and ECV contraction or expansion, or the presence of blood in the gut.

8. List five reversible conditions that can aggravate renal failure.

Hypertension

Obstruction

Nephrotoxins

Infections

Hypoperfusion

9. **List the most important factors in bone metabolism in patients with chronic renal failure.**

Phosphate retention

Hypocalcemia

Active vitamin D deficiency

Hyperparathyroidism

Index

Page numbers followed by an *f* or *t* indicate figures and tables respectively.

Page numbers followed by an *f* or *t* indicate figures and tables respectively.

Page numbers followed by an *f* or *t* indicate figures and tables respectively.

Page numbers followed by an *f* or *t* indicate figures and tables respectively.
